graceful
exit

graceful exit

HOW TO ADVOCATE EFFECTIVELY,
TAKE CARE OF YOURSELF,
AND BE PRESENT FOR THE
DEATH OF A LOVED ONE

GUSTAVO FERRER, MD
WITH KAREN CHERNYAEV

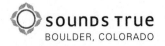

sounds true
BOULDER, COLORADO

Sounds True
Boulder, CO 80306

Published 2018

This book is not intended as a substitute for the medical recommendations
of physicians or other health-care providers. Rather, it is intended to offer
information to help the reader cooperate with physicians and health-care
providers in a mutual quest for optimum well-being. We advise readers to carefully
review and understand the ideas presented and to seek the advice of a qualified
professional before attempting to use them. The stories in this book are based on
real events. Names and details have been changed to protect identities.

Cover design by Karen Polaski
Book design by Beth Skelley

Cover image © Inara Prusakova
Printed in Canada

Library of Congress Cataloging-in-Publication Data
Names: Ferrer, Gustavo, author. | Chernyaev, Karen, 1961- author.
Title: Graceful exit : how to advocate effectively, take care of yourself,
    and be present for the death of a loved one / Gustavo Ferrer, MD,
    with Karen Chernyaev.
Description: Boulder, CO : Sounds True, 2018. | Includes bibliographical
    references.
Identifiers: LCCN 2017035186 (print) | LCCN 2017044470 (ebook) |
    ISBN 9781683640455 (ebook) | ISBN 9781683640448 (pbk.)
Subjects: LCSH: Terminal care. | Terminally ill. | Terminally ill—Family
    relationships. | Death—Psychological aspects. | Bereavement.
Classification: LCC R726.8 (ebook) | LCC R726.8 .F469 2018 (print) |
    DDC 616.02/9—dc23
LC record available at https://lccn.loc.gov/2017035186

10 9 8 7 6 5 4 3 2 1

To my beloved patients,
from whom I continue to glean
wisdom and knowledge

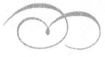

We may not ever understand why we suffer or be able to control the forces that cause our suffering, but we can have a lot to say about what the suffering does to us and what sort of people we become because of it. Pain makes some people bitter and envious. It makes others sensitive and compassionate. It is the result, not the cause, of pain that makes some experiences of pain meaningful and others empty and destructive.

HAROLD KUSHNER
When Bad Things Happen to Good People

Contents

Death Is Not Failure

Every day, at least one of my patients dies. Although that may not sound like a track record I should admit to, it's actually considered normal. Most of my practice as a critical care physician and pulmonologist working in the intensive care unit (ICU) in the Miami area involves serving those who are in their final weeks or even days. Although my team has succeeded in dropping the mortality rate below the national rates for long-term critical care patients, every day I'm on duty, I witness not only the loss of life but the familial aftermath—the shock, the tears, the screams, and even the cursing. Mostly, I see the confusion.

"Do you want me to call someone?" is usually my first question. Some people have me phone an estranged sibling. Others have me contact the deceased's spouse or another who is close and involved and often highly emotional. Almost everyone has me call someone. I am more than willing to do it. My firm belief is that empathy at the core of health care requires this action. I wouldn't have it any other way.

I didn't always feel this way. In fact, when a patient died, I used to feel like a failure. My training in Cuba taught me that medicine was the answer, and if a patient died, it was because I did not do my job.

I've since learned that death is a part of life, and the biggest failure is not death, but refusing to get involved in the process of dying. I've learned that dying ultimately involves the living, and so I make a point to help those who will soon be left behind make difficult end-of-life decisions, and afterward, I lend a hand when they are too full of grief to make a phone call.

I learned the importance of getting involved through the many family members who have entrusted me with the care of their loved one. Some of my lessons were hard, even shameful. Like when I was a young physician and Doris, a gracious, intelligent, and peaceful woman in her eighties, sat me down, as if I were her son. She gently counseled me about how devastating it was to her and her daughter when I, in my haste, jumped to false conclusions. Or when Margarita, after learning that her husband of forty-five years had died, looked at me, her eyes filled with utter confusion. Up until then, I hadn't taken much notice of what happened after a patient died. But Margarita triggered something in me.

Ever since then, I've been asking family members whether they want me to call someone. I keep making this small gesture because I've found that it goes a long way. These lessons and many, many more have left their mark on me over the past twenty years. And so now my practice is just as much about helping a patient's family members and friends as it is about treating the patient.

In some ways, this portion of my training came early, during the 1970s and 1980s, when I was growing up in Cuba. We Cubans are a passionate people. Family is first. The small farming community where I grew up lacked the economic resources and technology needed to prolong life. When, at the age of 102, my grandfather was dying of pneumonia, we did what we could to make him comfortable and accepted that death was imminent. We didn't have to consider whether we should rush him to the emergency department, increase his medication, or administer cardiopulmonary resuscitation (CPR). Without those distractions, we were present enough to feel our pain and lovingly tend to Grandfather. The family gathered, so about fifteen of us were around to help and support one another, as humans throughout the world have done throughout time.

Yet this is in sharp contrast to today's environment, especially in industrialized countries, where technology can dominate in end-of-life care and dramatically alter the experience. I've witnessed many family members instinctively, and sometimes out of guilt, make rash decisions to keep an elderly loved one alive by demanding certain procedures, regardless of how painful or futile they might be for the patient. CPR keeps the ninety-year-old with stage 4 lung cancer breathing, but it's painful, as it can break ribs and damage muscles and skin, causing stabbing chest pain. Pain and bruises result from the needles needed to access veins. A feeding tube inserted through the mouth or nose can stimulate the gag reflex and trigger vomiting. These scenarios are commonplace, almost everyday occurrences in almost every hospital in America. Although a blessing on many fronts, advancements in medicine can make acceptance of the inevitable harder for everyone, including ICU medical staff, who cite dealing with family members as the number one reason for burnout.

And that is how I came to write this book. We live in the Information Age, but no one seems to know what to do before, during, or after a family member becomes terminally ill, whether with cancer, heart disease, or dementia. As the technology behind health care keeps improving, our notion of how to interact with it on a human level is at times nonexistent. We are in uncharted territory. Families are torn. Doing what is available to them translates into doing what is right. But this is not always the case. This is only one of the reasons families need help from the clinicians and staff who serve the patient. I and every other ICU clinician repeatedly witness the same scenarios. We can almost predict when conflict will erupt among family members wrought with grief. We sense when emotions will trigger irrational decisions or behavior. Families have the medical facts, the advice of doctors and other medical staff, and sometimes family and friends, yet they hold on to the belief that twenty-first-century medicine will pull their loved one through.

Because of what I witness through my practice, I feel compelled to communicate three important messages: First, death is not failure. Aggressively treating the patient who has a chance of surviving is our responsibility but so is recognizing when the patient is no longer helped by modern medicine. Pretending otherwise is hubris.

Second, family members of a dying patient deserve guidance, respect, and compassion. For many people, dying is no longer simple, like it was for my grandfather. The impact of a family's decisions is more complicated than it was even thirty years ago. Clinicians know the drill. Most family members do not. Hospital staff has a responsibility to help people put it all into perspective.

Lastly, the behaviors and decisions of family members and medical staff play a large role in determining whether a patient leaves this world with grace and dignity. For the sake of the patient, we must all allow our moral compass to guide us, to be fully human during this most spiritual of experiences.

I see death more often than most people, but death is a part of everyone's life at one point or another. And when it touches us, it has the power to change us, like it did me, regardless of which side of the bed we're sitting on.

The New Rules of Dying

Modern medicine, specifically hospital medicine, has in recent years changed the way we die. *Consequently, most people are in the dark when it comes to knowing how to manage the end-of-life decisions that are now upon us—the ones that sometimes need to be made quickly in an ICU, as well as those we have time to prepare for.* Graceful Exit is a conversation about how to die, and let others die, with grace and dignity in this age of modern medicine. It's also a plea to make expressing end-of-life wishes as common as sharing what's on your Christmas list, what kind of cake you want for your birthday, or what you want for supper.

In some ways, this book answers the question: Is there a right way to die? The answer is yes, with a caveat—the right way is different for everyone. *Graceful Exit* sets a framework for how to approach a loved one's death with an elevated sense of responsibility and compassion. It asks us to acknowledge the deeply buried and sometimes overwhelming emotions that surface when facing loss and to use them as a bridge to a higher love. Loss, instead of being a source of pain, paralysis, and conflict, becomes a vehicle for knowing how connected we all are—with those we can easily love, as well as with those we harbor resentments against. Loss takes us out of ourselves, even as we reach inward. It forces surrender, acceptance, and with any luck, forgiveness. Rather than try to understand death, we surrender to it. We fall *into* grace, knowing we cannot fight death forever.

This book is intended to help you—a family member of a chronically or terminally ill patient, a parent who wants to get advance directives and inheritance documents in order for her children, a recent widower who has no idea what to do next, or a clinician who is interested in more fully understanding the patient experience—comprehend the new rules of end-of-life medical care: the advantages, the limits, the necessary preparations, the roles family members must play, the responsibilities of medical teams, and the cost considerations. We cover the nuts and bolts, such as the importance of advance directives and who to contact after someone dies, as well as some of the bigger ethical issues: do we prolong death using painful interventions that will buy the patient a bit of time, or do we, in spite of our capabilities, let nature take its course?

One beautiful Saturday morning last year I was supposed to be at the wedding of a dear friend, but instead I found myself in the emergency room, frantically performing CPR on Jane. Seventy-year-old Jane was visiting Miami from New York when she collapsed and could not be revived. She was rushed to the hospital where my team began working to try to save her. She was relatively young and healthy, but for some mysterious reason, she was bleeding internally, her heart had stopped beating, and her lungs had ceased to pump oxygen.

We tried everything to bring her back to life: standard medications, off-label medications, machines, pumps, tubes, and numerous procedures. Her husband, who sat in the waiting room during those tense few hours, added prayer to the efforts.

I am relieved to tell you that Jane survived. She walked out of the hospital several weeks after her ordeal with no lasting effects. She hasn't had a relapse, thank God.

Jane and patients like her are the reason I practice modern medicine. Not only do patients like Jane routinely make it through situations they wouldn't have just a few short decades ago, but many of the ills that once killed millions are now tamed to the point of near extinction. What we physicians can now do for our patients is nothing short of amazing. And the results grow more miraculous with each new breakthrough.

Another case in point: My good friend and retired physician, Dr. C, collapsed while having breakfast. His wife found him unconscious and immediately called 911. A specially outfitted ambulance with a CT scan in the back came to his driveway. The brain scan, which indicated a stroke, was performed and read by our hospital radiologist before the paramedics left Dr. C's house. On the way to our emergency room, he was treated with a clot buster, and by the time I saw him in the ER, he was back to normal. That's the miracle of modern medicine.

For patients like Jane and Dr. C, who are generally strong and healthy, modern medicine is at its best. But for the eighty-five-year-old with cancer, dementia, and a heart condition, the story changes.

Patients with little chance of survival—or at least little chance of survival with a quality of life—need a different kind of care. In almost any hospital in this country, a typical medical encounter like Jane's is handled the exact same way, whether the individual is 30, 40, 50, or 101. I argue that aggressive treatment does not serve every patient well. I'm not talking so-called death panels here, but I believe that we must bring some sort of sanity into the way medicine evaluates possible outcomes.

Hospital medicine's opposites are hospice and palliative care, whose main goals are to make a dying patient as comfortable as possible by helping to relieve pain via medication and offering emotional support and companionship. Most of the information in this book applies to all levels of care, from hospitals to hospice and everything in between. We will discuss hospice and palliative medicine, long-term acute care (LTAC), skilled nursing homes, and the growing home medical-care industry, as well as how insurance and predetermined limits of stay impact patients and family members.

We can weigh the good and ills of modern medicine till kingdom come. Modern medicine works miracles, or puts us in a difficult spot. The point is that it exists, and because it exists, most of us will come face-to-face with it at some point. And so I want you, the reader, to know some of the issues you will have to face and to have a method to deal with them. With this knowledge and perspective, you can go through the process confidently, centered, and at peace knowing that you have done due diligence for your ill loved one, your family, and yourself.

Everything starts with relationships. And perhaps never are they so impassioned than in an ICU. And so I begin this book with a chapter on what happens to family dynamics when on the brink of change.

Getting Everyone
on the Same Page

Rallying around a loved one in failing health can bring out the best in everyone involved. All too often, however, it brings out the worst.

In fact, one of the hardest things about a family illness is family. Heightened emotions, lack of sleep, and long hours of bedside vigil tend to magnify personality traits (for better or worse) and expose long-buried grudges. I've witnessed adults argue across the bed of a comatose patient, and I've seen otherwise sensible human beings practically come to blows over everything from who would receive certain items of clothing or china dishes all the way up to selling the family farm. It can happen with the sanest of families. Recently, my own family underwent a rocky experience over an elderly aunt's illness when people who were close turned against each other over a disagreement about how to manage her care.

I empathize with how easy it is to let ingrained dynamics and runaway feelings take over a situation. Yet when a family doesn't, can't, or won't come together in a crisis, the bickering or silence overshadows the critically ill patient's needs. Distracting disagreements occur at critical moments. It's draining and stressful—and almost always avoidable.

Relationships can be difficult in good times. Under stressful times, buried emotions such as guilt and resentment can emerge and clash, and we end up at wit's end, frustrated at everyone's behavior, overwhelmed with our own feelings, and lost in terms of how to handle it. That's why I chose to begin this book by exploring what's behind the family drama that surfaces when a loved one is ill and offering some ideas on how to manage it so everyone can concentrate on what matters most.

Understanding Family Roles in a Crisis

To better explain what can happen in the family dynamic during an emotionally challenging time, I'm going to use the example of the Rodríguezes. Angela Rodríguez was a widow whom I cared for over many years. She had four children—three daughters and a son. Toward the end, when Angela was diagnosed with advanced dementia and late-stage lung cancer, she was no longer able to speak for herself and couldn't participate in her own medical-care decisions. Finally, she was admitted to the hospital for what was clearly the last time. Her family gathered.

The youngest daughter, Maria, lived in New York, far from her mother's home in Florida. She hadn't seen Mom in several years and rarely checked in with other family members about Angela's health. Maria wasn't up-to-date on her mother's condition before she arrived, nor was she entirely clear about what was going on with her care. But that didn't stop Maria from swooping in and attempting to take control.

Maria harassed her siblings, barked orders at the nurses, and argued with me and the rest of Angela's medical team. She strenuously disagreed with every decision we made and was anything but shy about voicing her opinion. When the medical team recommended palliative care and hospice, Maria demanded her mother undergo a battery of what the rest of us knew were unnecessary tests. She insisted on ordering procedures Angela wouldn't likely survive and, according to her siblings, their mother wouldn't want. The rest of the family members were trying to hasten their mother's death so that they could inherit her money, Maria asserted. As for the doctors and hospital, she threatened to sue us for incompetence.

Experts have a name for Maria's behavior. They call it the "Daughter from California" syndrome. Compared to the rest of her family, the Daughter from California usually has the least understanding about what is happening to a loved one and carries the greatest burden of guilt. Unraveling everything that's already in place is her way of taking charge and channeling her difficult emotions.

The Daughter from California isn't always the youngest daughter, like Maria. For that matter, she isn't always female. She can be a mother, a son, a cousin, an aunt, an uncle, or a longtime friend. And she doesn't literally have to be from California. If we place this scenario in California, she can be the Daughter from New York, the Daughter from Kentucky, the Daughter from Ohio, or the Daughter from Australia. In my experience, the farther away she lives from the patient and the longer she's been out of touch, the heavier her conscience and the louder and more irrational she becomes.

The Daughter from California syndrome was first documented in 1991 by Dr. David Molloy in an article published with some colleagues in the *Journal of the American Geriatrics Society*.[1] The person described in this piece was the daughter of an incapacitated patient, and she did indeed hail from the Golden State. The descriptions of her tirades and tantrums are classic to any medical professional who has spent time counseling families at the bedside of a critically ill patient.

Janet, Angela's oldest daughter, had stepped in several years earlier to manage her mother's care when Angela first needed assistance. Janet lived only a few miles away from her mother. She was always the "responsible one," so she flowed naturally into the role of the "Leader" as Angela's health worsened. While it's admirable that Janet had done the heavy lifting of shuttling their mother to and from appointments, paying the bills, keeping the paperwork up-to-date, and otherwise maintaining a semblance of order in her mother's life, she sometimes got bossy with her siblings in a way they didn't appreciate. She took offense when they questioned her about her understanding of the clinical situation or Angela's finances, as if they were suggesting she didn't know what she was doing. This led to quite a bit of squabbling among the group. As Angela's condition worsened, clashes between Maria and Janet escalated.

Leader is a tough role to play in a family crisis. I have a lot of respect for anyone thrust into this position. Because they carry so much of the load, Leaders can sometimes resent the rest of the family for not doing more, yet they frequently feel entitled to make all the decisions, often without input from the rest of the family. In my twenty-plus years of practice, I have often witnessed leadership manifest positively. At other times, like in this case, the Leader is most effective at stirring up strife.

Jonathan, the second oldest and only son, found himself cast in the role of the "Mediator." Growing up with three sisters taught him a lot about conflict resolution, and it really came into play now that his mother was dying. Increasingly, he became the family go-between. As Maria and Janet's relationship deteriorated, he frequently stepped in to break up their arguments. For a period, the two sisters would only speak through him. It was very trying for everyone—including Angela's medical team.

Mediators like Jonathan soak up the emotional angst for the entire family. The effort to keep the outer peace roils their inner peace. Many Mediators I've known suffer from insomnia, anxiety, dramatic weight changes, and a host of other serious mental and physical side effects that result from the stress of constantly placating the family. In their efforts to keep the peace, Mediators often suffer more than any other family member, usually for naught. No matter how hard the Mediator works, the underlying family dysfunction doesn't change.

Finally, there was Samantha, the middle daughter. When Janet informed her that their mother's illness had taken a turn for the worse, Samantha booked a plane ticket to Mexico and didn't check in with the family. After about a week, a Facebook friend helped track her down, but even then she was reluctant to face the situation. Only after a brutal text and phone exchange with Janet did she agree to come to Florida and participate in their mother's care.

"Runaways" like Samantha can't cope with tough situations such as a terminally ill family member. I sometimes refer to this sort of person as an "Undecided" because of his or her inability to confront feelings or play any meaningful part in the decision-making process. Rather than pitching in, they are no-shows. Even when they are in the room, they are often reluctant to contribute in a significant way. They usually find it difficult to even sit with the dying patient. The idea of it horrifies them.

In many families, the Runaway is the most infuriating archetype of all, perhaps even more so than the demanding Daughter from California, the domineering Leader, or the martyred Mediator, who are, in their own way, at least trying their best. The Runaway's habit of checking out, especially when the going gets tough, can be difficult to comprehend. Others find it childish and irresponsible.

These types of family dynamics can surface at any time and place during the caregiving process, even in seemingly tight-knit families. End-stage caregiving can exacerbate them, however, especially if the patient is the last surviving parent or a child.

You might think that the Rodríguezes are at the extreme end of family dysfunction, but I've seen similar scenarios more times than I can count. But why does it happen? These siblings might not have been the best of friends, but they certainly tolerated each other, even enjoyed each other's company in other situations. Why would Maria make such a scene when it was so obviously detrimental? Why did Janet have to be so bossy? Why was Jonathan so weak and ineffective? And why did Samantha disappear? Did they not all love their mother and want to do what was best for *her*?

I believe that much of the conflict comes from a lack of empathy and understanding.

We can't always name our emotions or understand our behaviors, much less those of our siblings. Usually, we don't even realize we're misbehaving, and when another family member, in turn, reacts irrationally, we tend to focus on the unhealthy reaction, and the conflict escalates. We begin to treat one another with more and more suspicion, distance, hostility, and fear. The aggressive actions each takes toward the other are returned in kind but increased in intensity. Thus, in each round of exchanges, the parties become more belligerent, more hostile, and less cooperative. We speak of this dynamic as upward spiraling. Escalation, by its very nature, moves participants toward more and more painful conflict.

Naming the archetypes your family members are enacting can be useful in helping to interpret behavior, emotions, and reactions, all of which are personal but not always easily understood. They help put family dynamics into much-needed perspective. Having context can lead us toward acceptance—and from there to forgiveness and conflict resolution. Ultimately, everyone wants what's best for the entire family, most of all for the ailing loved one who may no longer be able to voice her wishes. To get there, we sometimes need to lay down our arms and follow our moral compass.

Moral Compass

When everyone's screaming, no one hears anyone. Instead, everyone's focus is on their own needs, pain, and confusion. In truth, it doesn't really matter what others say, how they behave, or how they communicate. A family member's irrational behavior only hurts our ego. It doesn't touch the authentic part of us, the grounded part that knows, regardless of the surrounding chaos, what is right and what is wrong. When the Leader is screaming over the phone at the Runaway for not taking her shift at the hospital, the Runaway's programmed reaction is to hang up and drive in the opposite direction of the hospital. But if the Runaway stops to consider what she knows is right—*that everyone in the family needs to pitch in with caregiving at this critical time and that it's important to spend as much time with Mom as possible*—she can take a huge leap and choose to overlook the Leader's behavior and do the right thing. In other words, the Leader's behavior doesn't change what's right or wrong. When we pause to consider our values, regardless of how others behave or what our initial reaction is, a peace settles over us. We know what we need to do.

Families that make an effort to engage everyone in the process—to ensure every family member's wishes, struggles, and concerns are at least heard—seem to get through the experience more easily. I see this over and over again. They are more present and better able to give their dying loved one the most meaningful care and attention. Achieving this sometimes requires distancing ourselves from other family members' emotional roller coasters and owning our own behaviors.

Changing someone's personality and behaviors is not an option, but we can change how we react to them and, in the process, take the relationship to a higher level. When overlooking difficult behavior is far beyond our ability at the moment, when forgiveness isn't even on the radar, and when personalities interfere with caregiving to the point of gridlock and exhaustion, talk to a counselor. Engage the entire family, if possible. A professional, third-party perspective is sometimes the best medicine.

End-of-Life Documents and Roles: A Glossary of Terms

Each state has its own rules and regulations regarding each of the documents listed below. To learn how your state interprets these forms, visit the National Hospice and Palliative Care Organization website at caringinfo.org, click on "Advance Care Planning," and select your state. All of the documents listed can be found online or via your doctor or lawyer and should be filled out when you are of sound mind and body. In all cases, the doctor in charge indicates when you are unable to make your own medical decisions.

Advance Directives. A set of legal documents used to state end-of-life wishes in the event you can no longer communicate. Advance directives may include a *living will* and a *health care proxy* (sometimes referred to as a *medical* or *health care power of attorney*).

Health-Care Agent/Surrogate/Attorney-in-Fact. The person you select to make decisions about your medical care on your behalf. A health-care agent may base his or her decisions on your living will. If the living will is outdated, the health-care agent, along with the medical team, may choose not to honor your wishes.

Health-Care Proxy/Medical Health-Care Power of Attorney. A document that indicates your choice of a *health-care agent*.

Living Will. A document that expresses the general extent of medical treatment you wish to receive if you are unable to communicate your wishes. A living will guides your family, health-care team, or health-care agent in making decisions about whether to administer life-sustaining treatments such as CPR, resuscitation, intubation, and artificial nutrition and hydration. You can request to receive these treatments if they will lead to recovery and normal function. You can request not to receive these treatments if they will prolong life with no sign of a return to normal function.

Durable Power of Attorney. A document stating whom you wish to manage your affairs if you are unable to do so. This person, called an *attorney-in-fact*, makes financial decisions but may not have the authority to make health-care decisions. ⪜

A Designated Spokesperson

On a more practical level, one thing that might have helped the Rodríguez family avoid acrimony is a document known as a health-care proxy. This legally binding document allows for the appointment of a health-care agent. If Angela had signed one of these in advance of her illness, she could have assigned one or more of her children the authority to make health-care decisions on her behalf as soon as she was no longer able to speak for herself. Besides giving someone else the power to make choices about her care, the document entitles that person to speak to her doctors and gather medical records without breaking any privacy laws. (The Health Insurance Portability and Accountability Act of 1996, also known as the HIPAA Privacy Rule, limits the amount of information doctors can give to patient families without a signed consent.) Ideally, a health-care proxy is part and parcel of a living will, which states preferences for life-sustaining treatments, such as CPR, mechanical ventilator, dialysis, invasive procedures, tube feeds, and others.

Filling out a proxy isn't difficult or time consuming. That's why it's so frustrating to me that so few people have them. A 2014 study published in the *American Journal of Preventive Medicine* found that only 26.3 percent of people have any sort of living will or health-care proxy in place. Respondents cited lack of knowledge as the most common reason for not having an advance directive.[2] It is possible that all the medical and legal terms confuse people. Worse, most people think they have to wait until they fully understand their wishes before assigning a health-care agent. The truth is that we all have uncertainties about what we want when facing the crossroads of a critical illness. Even with the best technology, we can't predict the final outcomes. And as technology advances, decisions about end-of-life treatment will likely become even more complicated, adding to the confusion. The more confusing the system becomes, the more we need help. We all need a trustworthy person to help make decisions for us when we can't do it for ourselves. Appointing a proxy you trust could be among the best decisions you ever make.

Life is finite, yet we celebrate the beginnings and run away from the endings. Filling out a proxy is an excellent antiprocrastination exercise, and it is extremely easy. It is not a perfect document, but it is the best first step. You don't need a lawyer. Most doctor's offices and hospitals have a standardized form they can give you, or you can download one from the Internet and file it anywhere you might receive care. (Keep a copy for yourself.) As long as it complies with your state's legal requirements, it is considered binding. Moreover, it only goes into effect when you are unable to participate in care decisions; if you regain that ability, the proxy gets tabled.

Obviously, the best course of action would have been for Angela to have signed a health-care proxy while she was still cognizant. Once she was incapacitated and without a proxy on file, none of her children had the legal right to make health-care decisions on her behalf, setting the stage for the ongoing sibling battles. When a situation like this escalates, it often winds up in court, where a judge appoints a conservator, giving that person the legal authority to sign documents, checks, and forms—legal, medical, or otherwise—on the sick person's behalf. (More about conservatorships and durable power of attorney in just a moment.)

Having a family member appointed conservator is a best-case scenario. In some instances, the court gives proxy and power of attorney to a legal representative or hospital administrator. It's safe to say that most of us would not want a court-appointed stranger making life-or-death decisions on our behalf.

It's important to tell the health-care agent you have chosen that he or she will make decisions on your behalf in case of incapacitation—and to update the proxy as your situation changes. One of my patients, Betsy, suddenly developed a debilitating disease. She became very weak and was not able to talk. She lived alone prior to the hospitalization and did not have children. A close friend, Toni, had been helping her for years, but Betsy had designated her only sister, Eleanor, as her health-care agent. The problem was that, following a nasty family dispute, the two sisters had not spoken for more than twenty years. Now Eleanor, the estranged sister, was in charge of making important decisions that were best suited for someone who knew Betsy better—someone like Toni.

I had a very emotional conversation with Eleanor, trying to get her to understand the position she was in. Nonetheless, she ended up authorizing unnecessary procedures driven by guilt, even though my patient had clearly stated that she didn't want to spend the last days of her life on machines. Unfortunately, she did, and all because of an outdated document.

Perhaps people don't talk about death and debilitation because in many cultures these are taboo subjects. But talk about them you must. You must believe me when I tell you that no family plan is complete without a clear statement about death and dying. If you have a family member whose health is seriously failing, make it a priority to get a proxy in place. Doing so helps avoid some very difficult arguments and disagreements.

Power of Attorney

Had Angela been lucid, she could have also assigned a durable power of attorney (POA) to one of her children or another party. This is a common procedure when a very sick person, often an older adult such as Angela who suffers from dementia or some other debilitating disease, begins moving toward a time when he or she will no longer be lucid enough to manage her financial and health-care affairs. In some states, a durable POA allows a trusted family member or friend to take the wheel on medical and financial issues when that time comes. In effect, it creates the conservatorship ahead of time, without having to battle it out in the legal system after the fact.

One important aspect of a POA is that the person signing it must comprehend the meaning of the document. This document protects the signer from being taken advantage of financially or otherwise, yet the person assigned the durable power of attorney could be held responsible for medical bills. Make sure you know what you are getting yourself into. Sometimes, a POA form is made "springing," meaning it only goes into effect when the grantor can no longer demonstrate the ability to make his or her own choices. In such instances, a physician must certify the person was of sound mind when signing the document. If possible, make sure this document is in place before the point of no return.

In Angela's case, she could no longer make her own decisions and could not at that point assign a POA. When a health-care agent or POA has not been assigned, the family must agree on who will be in charge of the decision-making. When disputes arise, the hospital has to involve the legal system. In the ICU, this happens more often than I would like to see. Fortunately, Angela's family realized that the legal route would be time consuming and costly, adding another layer of stress to an already stressful situation. Obtaining the proxy and conservatorship requires hiring a lawyer, setting a court date, obtaining expert witnesses, and filling out reams of paperwork. It would take the focus off Angela and drain their resources. Recognizing that this was not what they wanted helped them come together. They stopped fighting long enough to agree that Janet was in the best position to carry out her mother's wishes.

Communicate with the Doctor

Janet requested a brief meeting to ask me the best way to communicate with the medical team. When was I usually available? How often was it appropriate to ask for updates? And so on.

This opened up a clear line of communication between me and the family, making the flow of information and care directives much smoother. I was able to dial down the noise and deliver one clear message at a time. This helped keep the peace and improve Angela's care. Smart move.

In Angela's case, with Janet as the sole point of contact, communication was not only better, but it also provided a measure of clarity for the entire family. Having one set of facts, obtained at regular intervals, enabled Angela's children to move past many of the arguments brought on by confusion and different interpretations of the same facts. Although there was some grumbling among the siblings, Janet did a good job of asking detailed questions, taking notes, and promptly filling in the others about everything she learned. It didn't solve all of the conflict—believe me—but I did notice some measure of solidarity starting to form once they worked through this major delegation issue.

Seek Counsel

Angela's family ultimately admitted that they did not have all the answers and turned to the nurses on the floor for counsel and to help them confront the difficult decisions they had to make about treatment options. Janet told me that she viewed the nurses as a healing presence for her mother and siblings.

In fact, it was a nurse who suggested the Rodríguezes hire a personal care aide (PCA) for Angela. Angela's children would sit by her bedside for hours. Sleep deprivation and stress caught up with them, diminishing their capacity to think straight and manage their emotions. They fought the most when they were near exhaustion.

Nurses can only devote so much time to sitting with patients, so most hospitals and medical practices will provide a list of accredited PCA agencies through the administration or patient-services office. You can hire an aide for a few hours a day, overnight, around the clock, or episodically. A big advantage of hiring through an agency is that it takes care of scheduling, replacement staff, taxes, and all of the other bookkeeping chores that add up to more time and stress. I've seen some lucid patients object to having an aide at first. But they usually come around after a few days, when they see how much easier it makes their life and lightens the load for family members. Should the patient leave the hospital, the service can go with them.

An aide might help with basic daily living skills such as eating, dressing, and going to the toilet. Highly skilled aides may be licensed practical nurses, with the training to do tasks like drawing blood and administering shots. However, an aide's most valuable role is giving the family a break. Knowing that Angela was being looked after made it okay for her children to go home, take a shower, see their families, get some sleep. Relieved of some of their guilt and sleep deprivation, they were less inclined to argue. It's easier to come together as a family when everyone is rested and thinking clearly.

When You Need an Advocate

When a family is really having trouble understanding their options, or they are struggling to interact with the medical team, I recommend retaining the services of an advocate. This role can be handled by a family member or friend who understands the medical system and is willing to help, but other options are available as well. Case managers are on the top of the list, yet patients and families aren't always aware that they can solicit these services.

Case Manager

I don't know why case managers seem to be one of the best-kept secrets within the health-care system. Many hospitals now offer this service free of charge. Some hospitals and larger medical practices automatically appoint case managers in terminal or critical cases to hold your hand and advocate for you through a medical encounter. If one isn't automatically appointed to your family, request one from the administration office or check to see what options your insurance company will cover. If the hospital doesn't provide a case manager, the family can hire one, and in some circumstances, they are court appointed.

A case manager is a person or group with training in mediation and negotiation, particularly valuable when the stakes are high and fueled by emotions. A case manager's job is to look at all facts involved in the situation and make suggestions with the goal of reaching an amicable decision. They also coordinate insurance coverage, transition of care, hospice care, and prescriptions. A good case manager is especially helpful if you can't attend appointments or you're having trouble understanding your loved one's medical situation. Since they usually receive some training navigating the complexities of the health-care system, case managers can cut through the red tape faster than someone who has been newly tossed into the vortex of today's medical-care system.

I've seen some insurance carriers assign an internal manager to cases to help walk a patient and family through the maze of paperwork and procedures. Just keep in mind that anyone who works for an insurance company, however helpful, will probably protect the company's interests most of the time—that's just my two cents.

Social Worker

A social worker can be your best friend in a hospital setting. And their services are free of charge to patients and families. Not only do they offer counseling and support for the patient and family members, but they will ensure you have access to any needed resources. If necessary, social workers will attend court proceedings. They are also available to patients who do not have family.

Concierge Medical Advocate

Hiring a concierge medical advocate is one of the more recent options in case management. Concierge medicine companies are high touch and hands-on. Typically, you're assigned a skilled critical-care nurse or doctor who takes over everything, from looking over the charts to getting second opinions to making care arrangements. I've dealt with several high-end investment banks, hedge funds, and law firms that retain this sort of service for their employees and their families. It's a nice perk. Even if your employer does not offer you such a luxury, know that it's an option. Placing a concierge on retainer can run more than

$10,000 per year, with none of the cost covered by insurance. However, prices are coming down as these companies realize it isn't just the super-rich who need help navigating the health-care system. If you can afford it, the concierge approach is a high-quality help option. Be mindful, however, to get additional input if the service recommends unnecessary, high-cost interventions. Another solution is to hire a mediator or coach.

Mediator or Coach

Sometimes the type of advocacy a family needs comes in the form of mediation, someone to help them make decisions peacefully. A mediator or coach is not a preacher, teacher, judge, or mechanic. A mediator is not there to fix anyone. A mediator simply facilitates the conversation. He or she must try to understand what is in the heart of all participants, even if they don't see things eye to eye. The emotions flex the heart. Understanding a person's regrets, guilt, and pain will set the stage for civilized conversations. A mediator is a bridge who facilitates peaceful interactions. The mediator or coach must remain calm, be capable of controlling emotions, minimize gestures, be able to listen and remain neutral, and avoid agreeing with one side or a person right from the start. He or she can verbalize an opinion and then pause to allow time for others to speak. The mediator or coach should compassionately guide the conversation to reach an agreement or point of action.

To date, hospitals do not provide the services of a mediator on-site, but I am an advocate of having one on staff. The need for this service is high, and having someone on hospital grounds would be beneficial all around—to patients, medical staff, and families.

Angela's Final Plan

In the end, Angela's children came together. They were able to look beyond their differences and unite as a family for their mother's sake. The proxy helped. Appointing an official medical leader helped. Getting organized helped. Talking to the nurses and hiring an aide helped too. Now I want to share with you some other advice that enabled the family to turn things around.

Armed with her mother's proxy, Janet was not only a Leader, she joined her brother Jonathan in becoming a true Mediator. After carefully gathering all the facts about Angela's situation, she wisely held a series of family meetings to keep the family informed. There were still some tense moments among the siblings, but the family was able to agree on the basics of care and decision-making.

Those *family meetings are important*—I can't stress that enough. They work best in person, but if that's not possible, try to at least have a phone or video chat that everyone attends. It gets all players on the same page, or at least in the same book. If you are a family Leader, I recommend creating a list of talking points to share, so you don't leave out anything. If necessary, make copies of documentation in the form of medical records and reports for everyone to review. Having these conversations gives everyone a chance to say their piece and ask their questions. Schedule family meetings as often as needed. Sometimes this means every day or even several times a day.

You may want to consider asking one or more of the members from the medical team to join the conversation. It might be easier than you think. In 2017, Medicare started paying doctors for case coordination calls to discuss complex cases and end-of-life issues with patients and their family members. When doctors and other medical support staff are good communicators, they won't come across as if they are trying to force you into decisions. They can answer questions accurately and provide context. When done right, doctors and other providers help families share their thoughts in an open, nonjudgmental forum and move past their concerns. They back up the family Leader with facts and empathetic authority, adding a layer of trust.

The Rodríguez family meetings were beautiful. They began with everyone sharing stories from their childhood. Jonathan brought some of the family photo albums to the hospital. They sat by their mother's bed, laughing, crying, and remembering. Leafing through family photos as they played their mother's favorite music brought them closer and reminded them why they were there. That's when the ice between them truly began to melt. By sharing, talking, and understanding, they got past the differences and came to a mutual understanding. Most importantly, they became emotionally grounded and seemed to have forgiven each other for their differences.

In my experience, forgiveness is the hardest part of dying. Many of us struggle to understand a response to a critically ill family member that differs from our own. For example, why would Samantha run away or refuse to participate in the conversations? Once the siblings started listening to rather condemning each other, Samantha was able to articulate some of her fears. She was frightened of losing her mother. Angela was the thread that tied the siblings together, she explained to her siblings. Would that tenuous connection break upon Angela's death? Samantha didn't understand much of the medical jargon and was too timid to ask questions. She didn't know how to constructively participate in her mother's care. This is why she ran away. Her sisters and brothers didn't have to agree with her actions, but they could—and did—work hard at forgiving her and each other.

How a person responds in a crisis depends on their unique stir-fry of temperament, experience, and emotions. You can't live in another person's head, but you can try to comprehend what they're thinking by asking thoughtful questions and talking it out. Setting aside differences and replacing them with empathy, forgiveness, and understanding is critical. Getting to that point is not always easy. I know how hard this is from my own experience and from dealing with families for so many years. But remembering that you do it in the service of your sick loved one can give it purpose and meaning.

Clearing the air enabled the Rodríguez children to move forward. Together they decided on a short-term, day-to-day plan that included managing visits, finances, and responsibilities. With the help of Angela's medical team, they agreed on a long-term plan for their mother's care too. Angela died peacefully surrounded by her children. In the end, they were all there for her—and for each other.

I wish I could tell you that doing everything right will get you to the same place as the Rodríguez family. As I have seen, it doesn't always turn out that way. Everyone is different, as is every family dynamic. But every step you take in the right direction will make the situation a little easier. Even if you don't get to perfect, you get to a better place.

ACTION   Ask Thoughtful Questions

If you can't understand a sibling's behavior during a family crisis, a simple conversation can sometimes open the door to understanding. It's important to remember that a person's behavior stems from his or her thoughts and beliefs. Fear-based thoughts cause negative emotions (anger, depression). Fears of being alone or lonely are common when a loved one is dying. Following are a few suggestions for how to get the dialogue rolling. One key ingredient is that the communication should be bathed in compassion. Other guidelines for this conversation are few, but they are important:

- Be present (no cell phones in hand).
- Listen (summarize others' statements).
- Do not judge.
- Do not react.
- Do not accuse.
- Look for what you can give (rather than take).

If having a conversation is too difficult, do your best to exercise compassion in your thoughts. Acknowledge where the behavior is coming from and accept that it is based on fear. When you feel ready to start the dialogue, consider one of the following approaches:

- I know Mom's illness is hard for you. It's hard for me too. What can I do to help?
- I don't care how angry you get. I still love you and always will. I want you to know that, no matter what happens, everything will be okay.
- The best gift we can give Mom today is the gift of unity. Can I hug you?
- I know Mom is waiting for this . . . will you forgive me?

Caring for You

As you take this journey with your loved one, don't forget about yourself. You need to honor the fact that you are a mere flesh-and-blood mortal who can only go so far on little sleep and rampant emotions. Clear your mind when you can. Walk, take deep breaths, and find a quiet corner to decompress. Any reasonable chance you have to remove yourself from a heated family situation can help reset your composure.

Main Chapter Takeaways

- Understand each family member's role for insight into his or her thoughts, emotions, and behaviors.

- Get a health-care proxy in place, preferably one that includes a living will that gives a family member the right to make medical decisions.

- Appoint one family liaison, preferably the proxy, to be the point person with the medical team.

- Cultivate support in the form of nurses, aides, navigators, and advisers. If need be, hire an aide or consultant.

- Keep records and take notes. You can distribute these to the medical team and to family members.

- Have family meetings to discuss short-term plans and long-term goals of care.

- Practice forgiveness and understanding for the sake of your loved one.

- Take care of yourself by sleeping, eating well, and reducing stress. It's much harder to make decisions or negotiate when you don't feel your best.

Letting Head and Heart Guide You Through the Hardest Decisions

Translated from Latin, *deus ex machina* means "a god from a machine." In ancient Greek and Roman plays, the phrase referred to a crane that held the image of a god above the stage, a power introduced to suddenly solve a problem the play's characters had been struggling with. In today's world, the godlike machines sit in hospitals. Instead of cranes, they are catheters, respirators, and any assortment of tubes necessary to support life. The problem they solve is not whether boy meets girl but whether someone lives or dies. And the story concerns the precious life of a loved one.

Making the decision to remove a loved one from life support is *never* easy. Many factors come into play, including age, number of medical conditions, and how much intervention is too much given the prognosis. Of equal importance is the patient's personal story—a desire to live to see a grandchild born or until a loved one can fly home. This story goes hand-in-hand with the patient's wishes—those expressed legally through advance directives, as well as those discussed casually with friends and family. Religious and spiritual beliefs may dominate among these factors. But in my experience, the power of a family's instinct often overrules everything.

A Family's Strongest Instinct

I recently cared for an elderly gentleman after he had endured a massive stroke. He was in the ICU, intubated for weeks and weeks. Despite all the antibiotics we pumped into him, his infectious complications grew. There was no solution. We could keep him alive perhaps a few weeks longer, but that was the best we'd be able to do.

As a physician, it is difficult to approach the family of such a patient. As terrifying as the tubes and wires and machines needed to keep the lungs billowing, the heart beating, and the body nourished are, quite often a family's strongest instinct is to keep their loved one alive for as long as possible, by any means possible, including by depending on the godlike hospital equipment for far too long. Yet as a physician, this I know: every day that a patient like this lingers increases the potential for suffering that comes from a worsening condition and from the medical interventions designed to keep him alive and breathing.

A well-informed patient or family is key to turning what can be the most contentious part of all life-and-death decisions into a sound resolution based on love, respect, and understanding. In the best of circumstances, your loved one's medical team will deliver this information to you with compassion. But you might feel overwhelmed and lost in a sea of data, beliefs, emotion, and advice—or struggle to get the information you need. In this chapter, I show you a way to get what you need in order to merge instinct with rationality when under pressure to make what is, without a doubt, one of the hardest decisions you will ever have to face.

All of us must exit this earth. In the case of end-of-life support, we have some degree of control about when, where, and how. If we subscribe to the idea that a graceful exit is in everyone's best interest (which, by now, I hope you do), our goal is to make our decision feeling grace and peace in our hearts. And so here is where science meets spirituality: a great deal of grace and peace can come from knowing and interpreting the scientific data, all while considering your loved one's values and personal story.

When making end-of-life decisions, family members must momentarily set instinct aside, at least long enough to weigh all these factors and discuss them with family and anyone else involved. When family members don't agree on a plan—which happens a lot, especially in the early hours at the hospital—even the most obvious action becomes a source of contention. So it's helpful to have some guidelines you can follow.

The plan I'm offering you here is a balanced approach between the two current trends in medical practice: one is full of overpromises resulting in overtreatment; and at the opposite extreme is a pragmatic view based entirely on quality of life and usefulness—if the person is no longer useful, dispose of him. A doctor may take one or the other approach or something in between. He or she will communicate these thoughts through words, actions, and body language. You, as an involved family member, will pick up on what the doctor believes. But regardless of what the doctor's fundamental beliefs are about life and death, we can start to reach a balance between these two competing ideas and come to our own conclusions. We can start by looking closely at the medical facts.

When the Best Medicine Hurts

Like everything we perceive as "good," advances in medical care can be a double-edged sword. As clinicians, we can keep patients alive long enough to give their bodies a chance to recover, so they can sustain themselves. But when recovery does not happen, or when the patient suffers from multiple life-threatening conditions, these advances in care cross a line. They can move from being a blessing to a curse. The patient doesn't get better but either drifts along or gets worse. Usually, these patients get caught in a treatment cascade, where the fix for one problem creates another problem so that discomfort and suffering escalate, often in the form of bedsores, broken ribs, and infection.

Using CPR to resuscitate a patient who has stopped breathing and has no pulse can result in broken ribs (an acceptable risk when a person has a chance at recovering), which causes pain every time the patient breathes, coughs, or otherwise moves. Patients who are connected to breathing and dialysis machines frequently suffer through the infectious process, which involves pneumonia, skin infections, and ulcers. All of this is complicated by low blood pressure, so we must use potent medications called vasopressors to increase blood pressure. They work by squeezing the blood vessels in the legs and arms. In many instances, the blood supply permanently ceases to reach the fingers and toes, resulting in dead tissue (an initially painful condition we call "dry gangrene," in which the skin blisters and turns black and blue). Once the muscles begin to deteriorate, most organs will shut down. The smell of dead tissue starts to colonize the patient's room. When we reach this point, the battle is lost no matter what we do.

Most ICU clinicians intuitively know when ending life support becomes the better option. They see the same scenarios almost every day. Families, however, only see another day spent with Mom or Dad. This is understandable and reasonable but only to a point. Relying on life support when efforts to save a dying patient only produce more pain prolongs the inevitable—sometimes for a day a week or a month, and sometimes for a year. And it hurts the patient.

Many families choose hospice or palliative care toward the end of life (see page 31). Still, it is not uncommon to see dying patients linger in a hospital, hooked up to machines and surrounded by strangers in a sterile environment. In some cases, the family members who chose to keep their loved one on support show up less and less often to visit. On paper, it sounds cold and cruel, yet it all boils down to perspective. Loved ones believe they are doing the right thing by keeping Mom or Dad (husband, wife, son, daughter) alive. They are acting on a primal instinct: survival is good. In this day and age when medicine is the *deus ex machina*, they have no context for believing otherwise.

For perspective, I'm going to share some true stories with you. The names and some of the details have been changed to protect the patients, but these are stories of real people I cared for in the ICU.

Mr. Nathaniel Abrams's Case

The Abrams family had been well known to the hospital staff over the course of a year because of the attentive and involved care they provided for their father, Nathaniel. When Nate first came to our hospital, he was eighty-nine years old with multiple medical problems, including diabetes, hypertension, and kidney failure. He had also suffered a massive stroke that caused severe, permanent brain damage. As a result of having spent months in bed, he had developed multiple decubitus ulcers, commonly known as bedsores, in various stages from blisters to wounds in the back that penetrated all the way to the bones. He also suffered from a lower left leg fracture, leaving him with one leg four inches shorter than the other.

I remember seeing his family (prior to our team being consulted for a second opinion), his two sons and his daughter, always by his side, day and night. I am almost always uplifted when I see family members tend to a loved one in the hospital, but I felt a different sensation with the Abrams family. To me, they seemed driven more by a false sense of optimism than by the reality of what was happening to their father's health.

They were often in the hospital hallways, pacing in and out of his room from early morning and until late at night as if they were sentries looking out for their father on the "battlefield." They were there to be their father's advocate, constantly requesting assistance from nursing or the nurse assistant to ensure he was turned frequently due to his pressure sores and that he was cleaned as needed. The siblings would sleep overnight at the hospital, each of them taking turns lying next to him, making sure everything was all right. The daughter kept a very detailed log of everything that went on during the months Nate was hospitalized. She recorded urinary output, medications administered, vital signs, new wounds that popped up, and ventilator settings. But I'm not sure how they evaluated the information they collected. The Abrams children had an immense, unfathomable amount of love, in an almost zealous sense, for their father. And I believe it was this devotion to him that prevented them from taking a step back to see the bigger picture: their father's health was only declining, albeit gradually.

Before coming to see us, Nate had been discharged from an LTAC hospital. He was initially discharged with the plan of entering hospice care. His family, however, rescinded this plan. Nate again went into another cycle of acute-care hospitalization and was then transferred to the LTAC facility in hope of recovery. During this second admission, however, he continued to deteriorate and went into total muscle fatigue, a condition in which the lungs are incapable of breathing out carbon dioxide. He was in respiratory failure. He was sent to the hospital, where a major decision had to be made: to intubate or not to intubate.

From Tracheal Intubation to Tracheostomy

The main purpose of intubation is to maintain an open airway and facilitate ventilation. Ensuring that an unconscious or traumatized patient has an open airway is a doctor's number one priority. If the airway is blocked, the patient can't breathe. Intubation can be temporary: A plastic tube is inserted through the nasal passage or mouth and into the trachea (windpipe). The tube is then hooked up to a ventilator, or breathing machine. Temporary intubation is appropriate for about one week. If the patient cannot breathe on his or her own after that, a surgical procedure called a tracheostomy is the next step. "Traching" a patient requires surgically opening the trachea through the neck to insert a more permanent tube. Risk factors include the following:

- Inability to be weaned off the ventilator
- Obstruction of the oronasal passages (in the case of burns, facial fractures, infection, laryngeal cancer)
- Inability to protect respiratory function (in the case of a massive stroke, head trauma leading to unconsciousness, or chronic debilitating neuromuscular diseases)

"Do Not Intubate" (DNI) orders overrule this step, precluding oronasal intubation and tracheostomy. A DNI order can be discontinued by the patient or proxy at any time in the treatment process.

⚘ DNR, DNI, and AND Orders

Medical acronyms can be confusing. The following is a quick guide to some critical ones.

DNR: Do Not Resuscitate. When a patient stops breathing or the heart stops beating, a DNR order dictates that clinicians are not to perform CPR—no chest compressions, cardiac drugs, or breathing tube.

DNI: Do Not Intubate. CPR and cardiac drugs are allowed, but a breathing tube is not allowed.

AND: Allow Natural Death. An AND order ensures that the only medical measures allowed are to make the patient as comfortable as possible (pain medication, for instance). Fluids, feeding tubes, and other artificial means of support are not allowed. AND is akin to hospice and palliative care (see page 31). ⟿

Tracheostomy is a major medical decision when a patient is unconscious with multiple debilitating and nonreversible medical problems, such as a severe stroke, kidney failure, heart failure, chronic bronchitis, or chronic circulatory problems responsible for multiple hospitalizations. As time passes, infections, nutritional deficiencies, and muscle weakness can create a downward spiral, and weaning off the breathing machine becomes more and more difficult. The chances that Nate would successfully come off the breathing machine were close to zero, given the extent of his brain damage plus all of his other preexisting medical conditions.

We tried our best to educate the family about what would be involved in extubating and weaning off the ventilator for a man in Nate's condition. It's a delicate procedure that can damage the vocal cords, teeth, and lips. It can also perforate the back of the throat, breaking the trachea (windpipe) or ending up in the esophagus (food pipe), an event that drastically lowers oxygen levels, resulting in further brain damage. The chances of complications from intubation are far lower with an elective surgical procedure or in young people. Their mouths can be opened with minimal limitations. Older adults and patients with chronic debilitating diseases are a different story. Arthritis and muscle rigidity are among the most common limitations for mouth opening. Even with this information, the family decided to go forward with intubation, still with an unrelenting optimism.

We performed the tracheal intubation. Eventually, Nate reached the point where the plastic breathing tube in his mouth needed to be made more permanent. This tube can be used for a limited number of days before it induces mechanical complications such as burning of the tongue and vocal cords. The tube is held by tape or adhesive plastic and can easily dislodge and come out—a relatively common complication in ICUs. To avoid this complication, we tend to keep patients sedated, which in turn contributes to the prolonged intubation. After a week of being connected to the breathing machine via the plastic tube, the patient must undergo the procedure again, this time with the more permanent version.

Nate required placement of a tracheostomy, a surgical procedure performed under general anesthesia in the operating room. In this procedure, the surgeon cuts the skin right below the Adam's apple to reach the windpipe and then passes a rigid plastic tracheostomy tube into the windpipe. A tracheostomy is not a complicated procedure for a generally healthy person, but this wasn't the case for Nate. His neck was short and wrought with severe arthritis, which limited the extension. He was also on blood thinners, which makes bleeding highly probable. We can easily put pressure and stop the bleeding on our skin but not on a windpipe.

Multiple attempts were made to wean Nate off the ventilator after he received his tracheostomy; however, due to his profound muscle weakness and multiple medical conditions, he consistently failed those attempts. The longer on mechanical ventilation, the more likely the patient will contract an acute infection, and this was inevitable for Nate. His body was simply not strong enough to fight an infection.

During the last few months of his hospitalization, Nate was in and out of the ICU battling ventilator-associated pneumonia, sepsis, and acute kidney failure. Despite Nate's declining condition, his family still wanted everything to be done. They became desperate and unreasonable in the sense that they did not take no for an answer. The family began blaming everyone for their father's overall deterioration and allowed paranoia to take control, even to the point of being aggressive toward hospital staff. They were desperate to the point that they were willing to transfer him to an acute-care facility and initiate an organ transplant to save their father's failing kidneys.

The nursing staff and physicians repeatedly approached Nate's family in regard to the sensitive subject of end of life. Our team spent hours educating his family about his condition and prognosis, attempting to get them to see the reality of their father's situation: He was suffering from multiple ailments and confined to a hospital bed without any quality of life. Each day, he became more bloated and developed additional skin ulcers. Despite having had endured some of the most advanced medical treatments available, Nate did not have any chance of recovering. His body was beyond repair.

Nate's last days were back in the ICU, where he stayed until his passing: in multi-organ failure, with severe septic shock, on life support, and with the maximum concentration of medications that supported his blood pressure. He was bleeding from the catheter placed in his urethra and from his abdominal feeding tube (PEG), mouth, and every orifice. His heart eventually gave way and stopped. After multiple rounds of CPR for over sixty minutes, the medical staff could not bring him back.

Nate had never made his wishes clear to his children, who in turn could not understand the limitations of medical treatment. I will never know the whole story behind their story, the reasons for their decisions. I'll never know, and who am I to judge? What I can do is teach patients and families about the limitations inherent in end-of-life care. I can also bring attention to the consequences of overpromising, perhaps one of the most common reason for the lack of trust in physicians.

Ms. Elaine Torres's Case

Elaine Torres, a sixty-eight-year-old woman, suffered a sudden-onset seizure episode and subsequent fall causing a massive brain bleed (subdural hematoma) that left her unconscious and with brain damage. Elaine underwent two emergency brain surgeries, including a frontal lobectomy, or removal of the brain's frontal lobe. Although a fairly common procedure for epilepsy patients who need surgery, the surgery, as you can imagine, doesn't come without risks or disappointment. Postsurgery, a CT scan of the brain showed she had already suffered from multiple strokes. The procedure showed no worthwhile improvement. Elaine remained permanently brain damaged, totally unresponsive (encephalopathic), and unconscious.

Given her history, chances of neurological recovery were slim; however, in the beginning of her admission to the LTAC facility, her family was optimistic. They took every little improvement in her mental status as progress and seemed very involved with her care. They visited her almost every day, more frequently in the beginning but less as time went on. They placed a stereo at Elaine's bedside, tuning in to her favorite radio stations for her to enjoy, and most memorably, they attached posters along the room walls, detailing her life and background, encouraging all hospital staff to treat her as they would their own family. This display was quite touching to all the staff. It elevated the sense of respect everyone had for Elaine and her family.

Throughout Elaine's stay at the hospital, the family maintained good rapport with the nursing and medical staff. We constantly kept in good communication with the family, updating them on any status changes of their beloved mother.

There were moments during our team's encounter where we felt as if Elaine were "waking up," brief moments where she would appear to mouth words or respond to her name being called. Those moments were short lived, as the next day, she would revert back to staring blankly at the ceiling with random, nonspecific head movements. She stayed like that throughout her hospitalization, with some good and some bad days, battling infection and recurrent seizures, transferring in and out of the ICU.

Over the course of more than eight months in an LTAC facility, the family came to terms with the fact that Elaine was not going to fully recover. Hospice and palliative care options were explored; however, her family was not ready to make that decision. Elaine was therefore transferred to a skilled nursing facility, where she lives as of this writing—occasionally visited by friends and family. She remains bedbound and in a vegetative state.

Hospice and Palliative Care

Hospice is a means for providing comfort and compassionate care rather than treatment or cure to terminally ill patients who are expected to die within six months. By entering hospice, patients or their proxies have chosen to turn down further treatment to sustain life artificially. A team of health-care staff and social workers, as well as clergy, ensures the patient and family have the necessary supports, including pain medication and a hospital bed (if at home), as well as spiritual and moral support. Hospice can take place at home or in an institution such as a hospice center or nursing home. With at-home hospice, the family must provide a full-time caregiver. The number of people choosing hospice care has grown in recent years, in part because the programs have expanded the types of diseases that can be addressed, including dementia and diabetes. Medicare, Medicaid, and most private-pay insurances cover hospice. In 2015, according to the National Hospice and Palliative Care Organization, a growing number—almost 45 percent—of deaths in the United States happened in at-home hospice.[1]

Palliative care is similar to hospice except it can begin at diagnosis and include treatment with the intention to cure. These programs are designed to help people with a serious illness maintain a better quality of life while they are undergoing treatment. Treatment takes place at home or through outpatient visits to the hospital, and a team of people visit patients at home regularly. Medicare, Medicaid, and other insurance providers cover all or part of the cost.

Analyzing the Data

No legitimate doctor wants to end a life prematurely or cause undue pain and suffering. In most cases, the information a doctor is giving you is in your loved one's best interest. The prognosis is not pulled out of thin air but based on experience and knowledge, with a dose of gut instinct. At the end of the day, however, doctors are scientists, and we turn to the available data to help us make life-and-death decisions.

To create a solid indication of your loved one's chances for survival and recovery, doctors use what's called an APACHE score. You may never hear the term when talking to your loved one's doctor, but you can be sure she's using it if the patient is in the ICU. If you're not sure, ask her to calculate it for you and to spell it out. Data may not seem to have a place in matters of the heart, yet the knowledge it relays can set your mind at ease, even more so when you are emotionally drained. Doctors find it useful to drive home the information to family members. It helps family understand the fine line between using technology to help or hurt. In my experience, family Leaders find this information extremely useful.

APACHE stands for Acute Physiology and Chronic Health Evaluation. Its use is standard in the ICU, where, within twenty-four hours of admission, your loved one's doctor should have the data in hand, ready to discuss it with you at the meeting you request. The system uses points to measure key physiologies to get a sense of how severe the patient's condition is. It looks at levels of sodium and potassium, white blood cell count, body temperature, responsiveness, and more. It takes into account organ function and whether the immune system has been compromised. Scores range from 0 to 71. The higher the score, the lower the chance for survival. The score is placed in one of three levels. Here's a simplified version of the APACHE score in three levels and what each indicates:

Level I   < 20 points = 80%-90% chance of survival

Level II   20-35 points = 50% chance of survival; very critical condition

Level III   > 35 points = 80% chance of death

The APACHE score is not perfect. The data indicate chances for survival, but as you can see, there's room for interpretation. At level III, the patient still has a 20 percent chance of surviving. Here's where the art comes in. Your doctor's expertise, the patients he's witnessed in his career, his observations, his estimate of quality of life, and his understanding of the patient's wishes all come into play when he comes up with a prognosis. Your level of trust in the prognosis is directly related to your level of trust in the medical team. Hard facts are just that—hard facts. But when you know the team has your loved one's best interest in mind, you'll feel that the information you're getting is worth listening to. I can't emphasize enough how important this trust is to your well-being.

The Power of Faith

I believe in miracles, and I've seen my share in the ICU. So I never underestimate the power of faith to heal. People of faith believe in what they cannot see; they place their confidence in the hope that God can and will unleash His power to heal illnesses or families. They put their trust in God before doctors, and I am not about to argue with that. After all, I've seen it happen—patients who've recovered miraculously from massive strokes, multi-organ failure, tumors, and the infectious process, for instance, despite the data pointing toward imminent death. Most ICU health-care professionals carry in their memory bank at least one recovery that can only be explained as a miracle. My own daughter, Lauren, is my constant reminder that faith has the power to heal. Her birth turned me from an atheist into a believer.

Lauren's Story

I remember vividly the day my wife, Nikki, told me she was pregnant. What wonderful joy I felt! But my joy lasted only twelve weeks, at which point an ultrasound revealed the presence of a placental tumor. At that moment, a deep pain conquered my heart, stopping it for what felt like several seconds. It was fear, of course; fear for my wife and for that little life inside of her that I began to love from the day I learned she would one day be part of our family. I spent hours and days researching all possibilities, which only seemed to add to my stress. Meanwhile, my beloved wife anchored her life in her faith. She was surrounded by a group of wonderful women from her church, who prayed for her regularly and visited once a week to pray directly over her and the baby.

Nikki was referred to the top perinatologist in Miami. We saw him every two weeks, and he patiently answered my hundreds of questions. At week 26, he found that the mass was compressing the umbilical cord, risking the baby's life. He sent the 3D pictures of the mass to many experts around the world asking for advice. Basically, there were two camps: some experts advised an early delivery, while others promoted a "watch and wait" approach. We all sided with the latter, with weekly follow-ups to check the mass and general well-being. At week 27, the ultrasound revealed that the baby had stopped growing. I could not sleep for a week. My wife, however, carried an incredible peace. We celebrated a few ounces of growth on week 28, but by week 29 the mass was as big as the baby.

The worry shifted to cesarean or natural birth, and with the help and guidance of a wonderful gynecologist and perinatologist from the Baptist Hospital of Miami, we decided on natural birth. On that day in June, after eight hours of labor, my wife anxiously anticipated meeting our daughter. I was expecting my daughter with much excitement and anticipation, but I couldn't separate the doctor from the father. I was also ready to meet "Mr. Mass," the one who had robbed me of my joy for months.

I was holding my breath. The baby came out first, and she cried, which gave me permission to breathe, laugh, and cry—what a confusing moment! Then I heard a distant voice, as if someone were speaking through a muffler, "Gus, Gus, cut the cord."

"Oh yes, yes of course."

Half of my brain was looking for the placental mass, anticipating problems and follow-ups. All of a sudden, I heard the doctor say, "Here is the placenta. Let's review this." I jumped and joined the review. Where is the mass? We moved the placenta around in search of the mass, but there was no mass to be found. I asked him to check again and again. Nothing was found. Nothing!

Some people may say it was false imaging, but the mass was present in *all* ultrasounds. Others may say it was a fluid cyst that erupted, but it appeared as a solid mass in the ultrasounds. To my wife, to me, and to our church family, it was a miracle. Lauren has been a healthy bundle of joy, a brilliant young lady who wrote her first fiction book at the age of thirteen. She is truly a gift from God—our little miracle who walks, talks, and loves.

I cannot even pretend to compete with God, nor would I want to. The best-case scenario is that God is working through me and every other clinician who must deliver a difficult prognosis. And so whether you place your trust in God or the doctor or both, my hope is that you can do so fully and then consider and honor to the best of your ability your loved one's wishes and values concerning death and dying before deciding whether to end or sustain life support. In the hospital setting, our job is to honor those wishes. Sometimes, however, doctors openly disregard a living will that crosses into a gray area.

Living Wills and Gray Areas

The living will is not a binding document and very likely will never be because it reflects an ongoing process. Although there have been reports of doctors disregarding a living will for financial gain, this is not a common practice. Doctors sometimes refuse to comply with the wishes reflected in the will based on objections of conscience or because they consider the wishes medically inappropriate. In these cases, the care should be transferred to another health-care provider, and the ethics committee should become involved.

It is important to review living wills yearly or at least when health status changes. Consider Mr. Aaron Johnson's story.

Mr. Aaron Johnson's Case

Aaron Johnson was a healthy seventy-five-year-old man with no significant chronic medical problems. After the death of his wife, he lived alone in the apartment he'd shared with her for nearly twenty years. I met him in the ICU with a severe urinary tract infection caused by the bacteria *E. coli*. Within hours of entering his body, the bacteria disseminated into his bloodstream, releasing toxins that caused a massive vasodilation with profound hypotension, a phenomenon called septic shock. He required a substantial amount of fluids and vasopressors (blood vessel squeezers) to keep his blood pressure within normal range. He became unconscious and could not keep his airway open on his own. His son, Eric, was by his bedside and showed me his father's living will. This simple document stated that Aaron was DNR/DNI. It listed no specifics, leaving no room for interpretation. I was not comfortable with this living will. Most living wills are not this cut-and-dried, black-or-white. Most are conditional.

I knew that Aaron had a great chance of survival if treated appropriately, which meant he needed to be intubated. Before offering my opinion, I decided to talk to Eric about his father. I needed to know more about Aaron. Why would he create such a vague document when it concerned life and death? I was searching for the story behind the story.

"What prompted your Dad to get this living will with no room for reasoning? You know, Eric, life is not black and white. Your Dad is healthy and has a great chance of survival. What was this past week like for him? Can you take me through it?"

"He is very active, involved in multiple volunteer activities. His life is full."

"Was he depressed?"

"No, no way. He fights against that. He is full of life."

After half an hour of exploring Aaron's life, I told Eric that I disagreed with the DNI. I was convinced that he had a great probability of surviving this event. The bacteria were sensitive to all antibiotics, the kidneys were slightly abnormal as a result of the low blood pressure, but the kidney function was gradually getting better.

"Eric, this is an area where medicine has improved tremendously. Most people in his situation survive, even when they have chronic debilitating diseases such as chronic obstructive pulmonary disease (COPD) or diabetes."

I suggested to Eric that he call for a second opinion. He called Aaron's primary doctor, who reviewed the records and called me. He had known Aaron for more than ten years and believed that Aaron would like to have a chance at survival. He talked to Eric and his sister. We all agreed to intubate but no DNR: if his heart were to stop, we would not consider doing CPR. Within forty-eight hours, Aaron had recovered his blood pressure, his fever was gone, and he was fully awake after I dropped the sedatives from his treatment. We removed the tube, and Aaron was back to normal!

Eric and I were at the bedside, and we waited until Aaron was fully awake to talk. I described the ordeal and confusion. He was glad we did it. He told me, "Doc, I don't want chest compressions, but a chance of survival . . . absolutely. I still have things to do on this side of the world."

The Human Element

You've got the data. You may have said your prayers. Now you need to look into your loved one's heart. Knowing what your loved one wants or doesn't want in his or her final days isn't always crystal clear. If advance directives exist, we owe it to our loved ones to abide by their wishes when it makes sense. When advance directives don't exist—or are grossly outdated—we need to draw from what we know about our loved one:

- Is he religious?

- What would his faith tell him to do?

- Does he value independence above all else?

- Would he be happy being alive but not "living"?

Sometimes, when family members gather at the hospital and begin to talk about it openly, they remember a comment here or a comment there that the patient made regarding how she wanted to be treated during the final days. These clues, small as they may be, help families form decisions.

The temptation to draw from our own beliefs and values is powerful. A daughter who believes in doing everything possible for as long as possible might face opposition from her father, who has seen his wife suffer far too long. When the natural instinct is to keep someone alive no matter what, I find that it's sometimes important to give family members permission to let go. I tell families they don't have to decide today, and then I prepare them for the flood of emotions. I spell it out. I let them know that guilt, anger, fear, confusion, and blame are normal human responses to loss. These intense emotions can blind us, and the simple act of carefully bringing them into the conversation is all a family needs to open the eyes of their hearts.

There's a time when you have a responsibility to keep fighting for your loved one and a time when it's best to let go. Crossing that line is not easy. No one can make the decision itself—what seems like a decision to play God—easier for you, but your medical team can help guide you to a place where you and your family are at peace with the decision you do make.

I have learned that people understand pain and suffering very well. When families grasp that, and understand that everything possible has been done, the decision usually just happens. People get a sense of relief when they make these kinds of decisions. It's beautiful and peaceful to see families reach this conclusion, where guilt is discarded and frustration is out of the picture and people just get down to the very essence of being a human and connecting with their loved ones.

The Decision to Begin Life Support

Many factors affect the decision to begin life support with a breathing machine. Mechanical ventilation is indicated when the patient's spontaneous breathing (ventilation) is inadequate to sustain life. The medical indications for life support should not be interpreted in isolation but in the context of each patient. Age, presence of multiple medical problems, and physical fitness will impact the recovery and prognosis of each patient. The following are reasons to begin life support:

- Persistent decrease in breathing rate (bradypnea [< 8 breaths per minute]) or total cessation of respiration (apnea) associated with respiratory arrest
- Acute lung injury (inflammation) due to infections, response to surgery, or complications of it
- Persistent fast breathing rate (tachypnea [>30 breaths per minute])
- Persistent low oxygen levels (<85 percent) associated with bradypnea or tachypnea
- Respiratory arrest after massive strokes, accidents, drug reactions, toxic exposure, or massive allergic reaction
- Gradual deterioration of breathing mechanics (tachypnea or bradypnea) after loss of consciousness from strokes, accidents, drug toxicity, etc.
- Respiratory muscle (diaphragm and chest wall muscle) fatigue
- Obtundation (a dulling or slowing of mental alertness that can evolve to coma if untreated) or coma
- Persistent low blood pressure (hypotension) with abnormal breathing mechanics (tachypnea or bradypnea)
- Acute or chronic nerve muscle diseases (neuromuscular disease) resulting in severe muscle weakness
- Heart failure with massive fluid in the lungs (pulmonary edema), which occurs when the heart is not capable of pumping the demands for blood supply, resulting in fluid accumulating in the lungs ☙

ACTION Connect with Your Loved One

Overwhelming thoughts and feelings have a way of sorting themselves out on paper. Take some time to answer the following questions about your loved one's health and values:

- What are the medical facts concerning your loved one's medical condition?

- What are his or her religious or spiritual beliefs about death and dying? If you've never discussed this, write down what you think they might be.
- What do you think the patient would do if he or she were able to decide?
- What would you want or expect your loved ones to do if you were in a similar situation?

Caring for You

Find a good listener, whether a nurse, care coordinator, friend, hospital social worker, or clergyperson. Look for someone who will hear out your side of the story without judgment and give you an outside perspective. Once you find such a person, try to articulate not only the situation but how you feel about it as well. I always ask patients who seek my counsel if they want my advice or if they prefer I just listen without comment.

Main Chapter Takeaways

- Making the decision to remove a loved one from life support is *never* easy.

- Age, number of medical conditions, as well as the patient's personal story and values must be considered.

- The natural instinct is to keep the patient alive, no matter what.

- Having the medical facts can help us override instinct when aggressive medical interventions would do more harm than good.

- You have the right to be treated with compassion by hospital staff and clinicians.

Your Best Ally

Working with the Medical Team

It was 5:00 p.m. on Christmas Eve. I sat down in the ICU call room and took a deep breath. I was one hour away from signing over my ICU patients to the nighttime doctor, and one hour away from a much-needed three-day vacation. I closed my eyes to rest briefly, and within seconds I heard, "Dr. Ferrer, *stat* [come immediately] to the ER. Dr. Ferrer, *stat* to the ER." I seldom get called stat to the ER, which is staffed with very capable doctors. This call means trouble—serious complications. I ran down to the ER and found a sea of nurses, respiratory therapists, and ER doctors running from one side to the other. "Dr. Ferrer, Dr. Ferrer . . . room 7. Right here." I made my way through cables and IVs to find the ER doctor holding a mask on the patient's face. The respiratory therapist was squeezing the bag.

"Hi Gus, a difficult airway patient," the ER doctor explained. "I attempted a few times but could not get the tube in. I asked RT [the Respiratory Therapy department] to bring the video bronchoscope and to call you."

"Absolutely. Let's keep the head upright, open her mouth with a laryngoscope, and keep an oxygen mask close by her mouth."

In a matter of seconds, I took a deep breath, prayed, and unconsciously held my breath as I felt my heartbeat pumping in my ears. Thankfully, I was able to navigate the scope with the tube into the patient's windpipe. The team clapped, and the ER doc and I saluted each other with a high five. I stepped out to the nurses' station to gather some history on the patient. Andrea was an eighty-two-year-old woman debilitated by diabetes and heart failure, and very much loved by friends and family. Her two daughters were outside the room clutching their hands as they watched the ordeal with the breathing tube unfold. I introduced myself to them. They were crying and trembling and still gripping their hands so tightly that their fingers were turning white.

"She is stable now and on the ventilator—the breathing machine."

They hugged me and went around hugging the nurses, residents, and medical students, repeating, "Thank you, thank you. Thanks to all of you."

They told me about Andrea's medical problems and of her multiple hospitalizations. We then talked about her family. Andrea had five children in all: the two daughters at the hospital, twin sons living in New York, and a daughter living in Colorado. All of them understood that their mother was critically ill. She was found facedown on her kitchen floor by her daughter who stopped by after work. They didn't know how long she had been lying there. The last time someone had spoken to her was two hours prior. At this point, we still didn't know whether Andrea had brain damage from the prolonged lack of oxygen. We went over the test results we did have, and before closing our conversation, I asked about Andrea's wishes: "Does she have a living will?"

"No, Doctor," the two daughters replied in one voice.

I make it a point never to judge this response. As much as I'm an advocate for having advance directives in order, I understand that taking that step is difficult. In some cases, people aren't even aware that they can appoint a health-care agent, for instance. "Okay, for now, let's get to work. We still have to do more investigating."

I went back to the ICU for my sign-out. Ready to go home, I had a deep sense of accomplishment. I sat down in the call room one more time, closed my eyes, and took a deep breath, followed by another one, when all of a sudden a thought crossed my mind: "What if she doesn't wake up? How will they respond?"

Soon afterward, my colleague and replacement for the evening knocked on the door and walked in. We reviewed the status of each patient. Another handshake and out the door I went.

Before I knew it, my short vacation was over, and I went back to work in the ICU. I got my sign-out, and Andrea was on the list. Her condition had worsened, and she was not waking up despite being off sedatives. I walked into her room. The wall was full of taped-up thank-you cards, pictures, and handmade cards with kids' scribbles—"I ♥ U Grandma"—and "get well" balloons all over. All five of Andrea's children stood up as soon as I walked in; the nurses followed me. The family once again expressed their gratitude to all of us.

The Magic of Teamwork

When families and the medical team work together for the good of the patient, I always sense a bit of magic in the air. Even when the news or the situation is heavy or sad, everyone working together for the good of another human being creates an underlying feeling of joy. I relish this feeling in my work. It tells me I'm in the right place at the right time doing the right thing. This type of collaboration usually only happens when everyone involved respects one another. In my opinion, respect is a natural by-product of good communication. And good communication is a two-way street. When family members approach the medical team with respect, the team is more likely to respond in kind. So I encourage you to view the medical team as your ally and communicate with them—they are there to help.

In the hospital, the medical team is your best ally. Not only are they available for support and comfort, but at this point in time they possess the knowledge, insightful opinions, and important details about the current health of your loved one. Yet many family members are afraid to ask questions, aren't sure what to ask, don't want to bother the busy doctor, or go to the other extreme of ranting and raving and demanding all of the team's time. Procuring information is critical to understanding your loved one's medical state, and it begins with knowing what to ask—and knowing how to ask for it. In some cases, how much information you get depends a great deal on the relationship you have with the medical team. And so one of your—or your family Leader's—first goals after learning the prognosis is to engage the medical team by setting the stage for collaboration.

Appoint a Single Representative

In chapter 1, we talked about how Janet, the designated Leader in the Rodríguez family, took charge of communicating with me and passing the information on to her siblings. She set up a brief meeting to discuss the best way to communicate with me and how often. It worked. I find that it helps to appoint a single representative as an official medical go-between. Communications tend to be more productive. Your loved one's doctor can't process a blast of emails from one person, constant calls from another, and a barrage of texts from yet another only to deliver the same details about the same patient over and over again. It's a repetitive waste of everyone's time. Most doctors care deeply about doing the best job possible for patients and their families, and this means providing care and communicating. My preference is to do both well. But fielding the same questions over and over again is counterproductive.

Most doctors I know respond to messages as quickly as humanly possible—and the operant phrase here is *as humanly possible*. Sometimes we can't get back to a patient or family immediately or, frankly, in a timely way. So if a doctor doesn't respond immediately, try not to take it personally. Using Janet's approach to setting up the rules of engagement usually improves communications. Doctors know that the time they spend communicating is not going to be a wasted, or repetitive, effort. Most physicians are agreeable to reasonable terms.

If your Leader is able to develop a good relationship with the medical team, you are that much further ahead. Once trust has been established and you feel that you are being heard, the stage is set for good communication. When under pressure to make an important decision, you'll know that your loved one's medical team is approachable—and you'll feel confident they are giving you the best advice.

Collaboration Is the Goal

Ideally, the family's Leader sets collaboration as a goal. I routinely offer my patients' family members some guidelines about how to best approach their loved one's medical team. Over and over again, I find that this approach leaves family members with the feeling that they've done their due diligence and have the information they need to make their decisions. It also shows the medical team that you aren't going to drag them into a family drama (something they really don't have time for and that, incidentally, is the number one cause of clinician burnout in the ICU) but rather are interested in having a straightforward conversation. It starts with giving yourself time to think.

Nine Steps to Better Communication with the Doctor— Getting the Information You Need Most

1. **Assess the situation.** Unless it's a life-or-death CPR situation, give yourself time to think and understand the whole picture. Bring in friends and family to help you assess the situation. It has been said that those outside the chess game can see the play better than the players. If you have a large family, choose a few of them. Five is a good number. Too many can cause confusion and division.

2. **Ask for lay terms, please.** In your first encounter with clinicians, ask the doctor to describe the condition in lay terms. Don't feel intimidated or afraid! You have a right to know.

3. **Request a meeting.** After the first twenty-four hours, when the team has gathered information and lab reports, request a meeting. This first interview is to gather goals of treatment and encourage empathic communication that fosters trust. Being able to trust your medical team is essential. Request two things up front:

- Ask for a sit-down, private, face-to-face conversation. (If you cannot be at the hospital, schedule a meeting on Skype.) Sitting down relaxes you, and the clinicians will perceive you as not being in a rush. This encourages the doctor and clinical team's full attention. Tell them that you want specific information regarding lab results, other test results or procedures, and diagnosis.
- Respectfully ask your medical team to gather the opinions of other doctors and consultants.

4. **Openly acknowledge your feelings.** You may be feeling frustrated or upset. Openly acknowledge your feelings, so it's easier to set them aside for the moment. "I'm feeling frustrated and overwhelmed right now, but I want to try to focus on my father." This way, the focus of the conversation stays on the patient.

5. **Assess your clinician's level of empathy and compassion.** You likely know something about your loved one's values and beliefs. Share this information in one sentence: "He believes . . ." or "She never wanted to talk about . . ." Gauge the clinician's interest in what you have to say.

6. **Communicate the type of information you want.** Some people like details; others just want the highlights. Let the medical team know what you want by framing your questions appropriately: "Dr. Smith, would you explain the situation in detail?" or "Would you give me a general idea of the diagnosis and plan?"

7. **Understand the prognosis.** "Based on the information you currently have, what should I be expecting in a week, two weeks, months, years?" Ask them to explain any terms you don't understand.

8. **Summarize the prognosis in your own words.** Repeat it back to them and ask, "Is there any other treatment available?"

9. **Wait (if time permits).** Discuss with family and friends and, if you feel the need, call for a second opinion. It's important to process all the information, and that can take time. (I cover how to ask for a second opinion on pages 67–68.) ≈

Get to Know the Team

As I'm sure you know, the medical team is more than just the attending doctor and a group of specialists. There are always a number of other professionals on the front lines of care, handling the day-to-day needs of patients and their families. Relationships with these professionals are invaluable. Approach them the right way, and they will be your best allies.

Nurses are a constant in a patient's journey. In a hospital setting, they stay with patients wherever they go, knitting together knowledge of the person, knowledge of treatment, and knowledge of process. Close proximity often allows nurses to have a less formal and less threatening relationship with families and patients than some doctors might. People tell me they often feel the strongest bond of trust with the nursing staff. It's a nurse, they say, who helped them when they were overwhelmed with information and by the myriad of health-care providers they encounter, the fragmentation of the health-care system, and the many decisions they are required to make.

A good nursing staff can help you—and the patient, if he or she is lucid enough—express thoughts, concerns, and values. Depending on the facility, nurses sometimes have training in end-of-life care and end-of-life communication, giving them the skills to advise families of patients with a life-limiting illness.

❧ Names, Numbers, and Schedules

Make a point to find out the answers to the following questions:
- Who is on our medical team and who is in charge?
- Who are the two main treating physicians (that is, who is coming on the weekend)?
- When will the doctor be coming by?
- What number can I reach the doctor at if I have questions?
- Who is the nurse, the nurse's assistant, and the case manager?

These questions may sound simple and basic, but you would be surprised at how many people don't ask them. It's more than okay to ask these questions. You have a right to communicate with the medical team, especially with the one in charge. ❧

Every day that you talk to your doctor, you have to be positive and ask open-ended questions that trigger the doctor to explain more.

- Doctor, in your opinion, are we doing the maximum that we can do? What more should we be doing?

- Doctor, is what we are doing actually producing more harm? How so?

❧ Every Time You Communicate with the Medical Team
- Be positive.
- Ask open-ended questions.
- Tune in to the team's perceptions about the current level of treatment. ❧

You're not only looking for blood test results and other data. You want to be tuned in to the team's *perceptions* on a daily basis. The team regularly sees patients with your loved one's condition. Their perceptions hold some truth. You want to know if you are going too far. If you trust the team, you'll trust their responses. When I sense that people don't like or trust my answers, I sometimes encourage them to seek a second opinion: "You know what, perhaps we can call someone else to give you an opinion." I have done that, and I know many doctors who do that. "I think we should call this consult to get some expert advice." We'll talk more about second opinions later in this chapter.

If the Doctor Is Incommunicado

Some doctors don't bother trying to communicate well. In my opinion, they fall short on one of the most important aspects of their job—reassuring patients and families. If a family member of mine were under the care of such a physician, I would consider switching. A doctor who isn't a good listener and doesn't value dialogue, even if he or she is a fine clinician, adds turmoil to a family experience that is already difficult enough. If the doctor in question is doing harm on some level, even if only because of poor communication, consider finding a replacement. You have the right to do so.

Communication *among* Medical Teams

A word of caution: Don't take for granted that every physician on your team is sharing information with every other physician. In my practice, we have procedures in place to make sure everyone is up-to-date about cases. This is true in many practices, hospitals, and other facilities. This is also what should happen, and we always hope it does happen. But this is not always the case.

Communication works best among doctors affiliated with the same medical group. If a loved one's entire medical network is associated with the same hospital or large medical practice, it's much easier for providers to keep abreast of a patient's health status. Many groups share a unified record-keeping system, which gives doctors and patients access to all records in one place. When it's not possible to stay within the same medical group, then be vigilant about record keeping.

Ms. Diana Jones's Case

Diana Jones, a sixty-seven-year-old woman, suffered from severe rheumatoid arthritis, atrial fibrillation (irregular heartbeat), and chronic bronchitis from years of smoking. She had swan neck deformities of her hands (the joints of her fingers hyperextended so that they bent downward toward the palm; in Diana's case, the swan neck deformities were the result of rheumatoid arthritis), a short neck from compression fractures, and three toes that had been amputated due to severe circulatory problems. She came to the ER complaining of cough, green mucus production, a fever of 103°, shaking chills, and a worsening of shortness of breath. In the ER, she was diagnosed with pneumonia, and the ICU was called for impending respiratory failure. We treated her with antibiotics, fluids, nebulization (drugs inhaled as a mist), and oxygen.

Scott, the ICU physician on duty, called me to the ER to discuss her case. During his presentation, he held up a list of twenty-seven prescription medications, six over-the-counter drugs, four vitamins, and five "natural products" that she was taking. During the twelve to eighteen hours that she was awake, she was consuming forty-two medications—more than ten products every four hours. We dove into her records and discovered that she spent most of her days in doctor's appointments, and all of the physicians were giving her something. Pain medications, anti-inflammatories, anti-rheumatic drugs, inhalers, blood pressure medications, diuretics (water pills), blood thinners, over-the-counter pain medications, anti-allergy medication, antacids, and the list went on. Scott grouped the medications in categories that overlapped and then grouped them by side effects.

Diana's daughter, Cynthia, told me that Diana was experiencing nausea after starting a natural product for arthritis. The night before the ER visit, she took her narcotic pain medication (Vicodin) and went to sleep. Cynthia found her in the morning in a pool of vomit, conscious but confused. She called 911.

After learning about all of the drugs Diana was on, we determined that she very likely was nauseated from the medications to the point that she vomited but could not protect her lungs from it. How did we know this? Vicodin (as well as other opioid pain medications) can suppress the gag reflex and depress the breathing center.

Scott and I cut down Diana's medication list to eight pills. Three days later, she was up in bed with minimal shortness of breath. Diana was an unsuspecting victim of polypharmacy (the taking of multiple medications), which caused unintended side effects from bad drug interactions. Polypharmacy, not pneumonia, brought Diana to the ICU.

Limiting your loved one to twelve pharmaceuticals is a good rule of thumb, if possible. But regardless of how many medications and supplements she takes, you'll want to ensure that she is avoiding harmful drug interactions.

Medicine Checks

All drugs (including alcohol, prescription, over-the-counter, legal/ illegal) and supplements have the potential to interact with another drug or supplement and create an unwanted side effect or an entirely new condition. For example, when taken together, ginkgo biloba, a natural remedy for circulation, and Coumadin, a prescription blood thinner, significantly increase the risk of bleeding. Not all hospital systems are set up to monitor drugs prescribed by a clinic in a different system, and any system is fallible. So the onus is on you to initiate periodic medicine checks. Collect all medications from home, including aspirin, cold medication, prescription bottles, and supplements. Put them in a brown bag, give it to the doctor, and request a medicine check. The doc will enter the medications into a software program to determine whether any should be omitted or avoided. Continue to reconcile the list of medications the nurse gives your loved one: "What are you giving her? How long does she need to take it? Here's her current list of medications. I want to make sure it doesn't interfere with anything she's currently taking."

The Yellow Notepad

Maintain one notebook or file to keep track of important information. It doesn't have to be anything fancy. A simple yellow notepad will do. When keeping records, never assume. Missing information may be the key to getting the right care. Never forget that you are an advocate for your loved one. Keep copies of all records, and take the following steps:

- Make a list of all doctors, important phone numbers, and all medications.
- Distribute the list to each physician on the team and update it as necessary.
- Make sure someone is present to take detailed notes during each doctor visit.
- Request that specialists send copies of medical records to the physician in charge after each update and be sure to let each doctor know what has happened between visits.

You may have to follow up several times, so be prepared to stay persistent. Be polite but firm. This will annoy some physicians, but so what? A patient's daughter recently told me that she had to request a transfer of her mother's records five times before someone finally did it. Being an advocate isn't always easy. ✐

Bottom Line

A personal connection can do wonders during this process. Whenever possible, speak to medical staff in person. There is no substitute for gauging facial expressions and body language. Of course, if you are far away, this isn't always possible. Consider taking a few days to visit the hospital, so you can introduce yourself and strengthen relationships. When medical staff see that you're invested, you might be more likely to get a timely phone call and more information. After all, they're only human. If you can't be there in person, work hard to stay cordial through phone, text, and email, even if the person on the other end of the phone isn't reciprocating.

I wish I could say you won't encounter rude, curt medical professionals. I make no excuses for them. The vast majority of people who go into medicine tend to be compassionate and kind; most of them are helpful by nature. Whether it's the long hours, burnout, or the lower-than-they'd-like pay that erodes the empathy of a few, I cannot say. It is unfortunate when a patient or family member in crisis encounters people in the system who have forgotten their humanity. I once overheard a patient's daughter lecture a doctor she felt had been distant and vague about her father's treatment, reminding the doctor that he was dealing with a real, flesh-and-blood human being who only had one life. Could he possibly take the time to do more than order a few tests, she wanted to know?

When You Don't Trust (or Like) the Doctor

What do you do when compassionate communication is not on the doctor's agenda? If you and the doctor are having trouble communicating—whether because your personalities clash, you feel "unheard," she hasn't given you the time of day, you think she doesn't know what she's talking about, you sense the facility is outdated or poorly run, or you have a gut feeling that something is off—you won't be satisfied with what she tells you, even if she's number one in her specialty. I would advise you to either hand the reins over to another family member who can work with the clinician, take it up with a hospital supervisor, call in the case manager for help, or seek a second opinion.

Touching the Heart First

From the clinician's perspective, breaking bad news can be particularly stressful, especially if the clinician is inexperienced. I want to share with you a story of my own inexperience and the effect it had on my patient's family—and on me.

Years ago as a young doctor, I was called to the ER to see a patient in his nineties. He was coming from a nursing home. His blood pressure was so low that we couldn't even measure it. It was basically undetectable, a sign that either his heart was not pumping blood to his vital organs or the blood vessels were extremely dilated. His cells were dying. Soon, I was sure, his body would shut down. He was burning up with fever and dripping sweat everywhere, his body fighting infection. When I arrived in the ER, the nurse was waking him up so that I could speak with him. Although he was very responsive to my questions, he would mumble in-between. I knew nothing more about the case, yet found myself quick to judge. I started making comments with the nurses: "Why do we do this? He should be in hospice." While I was ranting away, the patient's wife, Doris, and their daughter walked into the room with trembling voices, trying to see what was going on. They approached me, and Doris asked, "Doctor, what's the problem?"

Without really thinking, I blurted out a string of medical terms. I remember that I told her he had sepsis and encephalopathy—I was using all kinds of medical terminology, and I was quick to verbalize everything that I knew at that point without taking into account anything other than my thoughts and frustration. I employed no filter, nor did I choose my words carefully. Instead, I went for the shorthand version, the dialogue that would say the most with the fewest number of words. I communicated a lot, all right.

"He's not doing well," I said. "I think you should consider making him DNR or sending him to hospice." In my haste, I rushed through my analysis and flooded that family with a shower of medical information without taking into consideration that I might be igniting confusion. Worse, I used an impatient and judgmental tone. I made no effort to conceal the frustration I was feeling, even though these two lovely people, who clearly cared for this man, were standing right before me.

Doris gently left and, with tears in her eyes, told me, "You know what? He will come back to me. I know he will. You keep your knowledge, and I'll keep my faith."

I didn't pay attention to Doris's words at all. Doctors hear these kinds of comments all the time. It can be easy to tune them out when we feel we have more important things to think about. Yet, when doctors are quick to judge outcomes, we run the risk of creating false expectations, good or bad. Doris, however, clearly had her own set of expectations, and at the time, neither of us were interested in battling it out.

Over the following days, our medical team gathered some information and did some blood tests, and I realized that what the patient was facing wasn't that bad. He was critically ill, but based on the APACHE score and the severity index that we do for a patient with severe infections, the probability of him fully recovering was pretty good. We put him in the ICU, and he got the appropriate treatment. The next day, I came from my rounds in the ICU and, surprise, he was sitting up in his bed having breakfast. You probably know what's coming next.

I walked into the room, and Doris and her daughter were there, and with a big smile, Doris said, "I told you that he would come back." I tried to do damage repair by explaining it was a false alarm initially, but after gathering some data, I knew he would recover. Unfortunately, the damage was done. I had lost their trust. After three days in the hospital—talking to them, being responsive, being there, not trying to justify anything—I was able to gain some ground in their hearts. By day five, the patient was ready to be moved out of the ICU to the regular floor in the hospital. On that morning, I happened to pass by his room, again in a rushed mood because I was in the middle of transferring another patient out of our busy ICU. I walked in to the room intending to give a quick "good-bye" and tell the family that he's doing great, but Doris wanted to talk.

"Come in the room and sit down. I just want to talk to you face-to-face," she said as she sat down. She asked me if she could hold my hand.

I said, "Sure, absolutely!"

She asked me to look into her eyes, and she continued: "Son, you have been gifted to help others. You have the gift of healing. Doctors have this gift. But before you make any comment, explore first, and never say 'never' unless you have the medical scientific evidence to back up your statement."

I acknowledged what she said, and after a little pause, she added, "You have to see that you are touching people's hearts first, and then you can engage in a conversation with them. But first, touch their hearts. Get to know them as human beings. They are not machines. They are human, they have families, they have needs, they have problems, and they have bills to pay. We are people in need."

I was listening carefully as she said, "You have to try to understand people more when they are walking through the valley of the shadow of death. Because this is the time when they really need less medicine and more compassion." She then looked directly into my eyes and said, "You don't have the final answer. God does. But he gave you the education you have to make an educated guess, a prediction. You have to use it right." She paused again for a few seconds and said, "Dr. Ferrer, this gentleman here in this bed, he was a professor of medicine and very well known in his college for forty years, and I was an ICU nurse."

Her words practically killed me. Five days under my care, and I didn't know that he had been a doctor, Doris had been an ICU nurse, and the daughter was a practicing nurse, and I made all of the mistakes that a young doctor can make.

Doris was a turning point in my life. She woke me up to the "other" important part of my role as a doctor. Right then and there, I made the decision that when doing my initial interview with the family, I would ask questions about family, friends, who's helping you, pets—to make a sincere effort to connect with the patient and family.

Doctors can have all of the knowledge, the science, the data, the statistics, but if we don't put compassion into the picture, we don't have the family's trust. If I'm going to have difficult conversations with families and propose gut-wrenching end-of-life decisions that bear any weight, I must have their trust. Having these conversations and making bold statements without having earned trust can be likened to asking someone to cross a frayed zip line with rusty gear. There's no assurance that the equipment is safe and secure. It's being flippant with someone's loved one.

We doctors save lives, but patients and their family members sometimes have the power to change our entire outlook when it comes to how we practice medicine. Do not be afraid to be a Doris. Be the person who holds the doctor accountable for not only delivering the best medical care possible but also for taking the time to touch your heart. Trust and acceptance come easier to family members when they believe the medical team cares about their loved one's welfare—when they know their loved one is not just a statistic, a chart, or a bed in a room. And acceptance is a precursor to peace.

Bedside manner aside, it's highly possible that the information the doctor is giving you is in your loved one's best interest, but his or her method of delivery is clouding your perspective. Yet, if you feel uneasy, do not hesitate to request a second opinion. I found myself in this position after my wife underwent a simple stress test.

Nikki's Beating Heart

My wife, Nikki, is a terrific runner, and if I may brag for a moment, she is so talented that she sometimes wins races outright—that is, she beats both the women and the men!

A few years ago, Nikki started complaining about a funny feeling in her chest every time she ran at a high intensity. When she slowed down, it went away, but it came back anytime she picked up her pace.

I was working hard and traveling a lot at the time, so at first I didn't pay much attention to her. "It's just reflux," I said. "Don't worry about it." But after a few days, something clicked, and it pushed me to make an appointment for her for a stress test with a prominent cardiologist I knew. I asked him to check her heart. "It's probably nothing, but let's just make sure," I said. He's an avid runner, too, so I felt he would understand where I was coming from.

He ran the tests. They showed nothing, but when I looked at how Nikki had been tested, I still had this nagging feeling that there was a problem. I felt they hadn't pushed her hard enough; she mentioned that she never broke a sweat or got to the point where she would typically feel the pain. I asked the doctor to do another stress test, this time a harder one, but he didn't agree. "She's fine," he said, clearly annoyed. "You're making too much of this."

I could have let it go at that point, but my doctor's instincts were now really tingling. I decided to go for a second opinion. I found another doctor who agreed to do the test the following day.

I couldn't clear my schedule on such short notice, so Nikki went to have the test alone. I will always remember getting that call while I was in the middle of a patient's exam. They told me there was something wrong, and I needed to come to the ER right away. The feeling of my stomach flip-flopping, then dropping into my feet, is something I will never forget. I got that call after Nikki's exam.

The second test revealed that whenever Nikki's heart neared its maximum effort, one of the walls in the chambers of her heart collapsed because of a malformed blood vessel. It's a condition we docs refer to as the "widow-maker" because it's rarely caught in time; most often, people are just walking along when suddenly their artery bursts. They die almost instantly. We caught Nikki's problem in time, and I thank God for that every day.

That experience taught us so many lessons, but the one I want to convey here is that you must be ready, willing, and able to stand up to your medical team if your senses start tingling like mine did. In fact, I encourage you not to wait for that gut reaction or your senses to tingle. There are questions you should *always* ask your medical team. The truth is you can love your doctors and not love their advice. They may get annoyed with you. Frequently they'll push back, and sometimes they may be outright hostile. There are reasons for these reactions—reasons deeply embedded in the medical system—but I'll show you some steps you can take to get those answers anyway.

The Fear Behind the Second Opinion

Many doctors react to a request for a second opinion because they automatically associate "second opinion" with "sue," and perhaps no other verb in the English language has done more harm to great medical care than that three-letter word. Doctors fear hearing it; frustrated or angry patients and family members sometimes bandy it about, and the word comes flying out of their mouths when they don't know what else to do to get their doctor's attention. It makes patients feel powerful, but most of them are saying it because they feel powerless. It puts medical teams on the defense, so much so that even asking for a second opinion can ring an alarm in the doctor's head.

So many doctors are afraid of being sued that the second opinion has become the Pandora's box of health care. It's a touchy subject. A lot of thoughts zoom through a doctor's mind: *They're going to sue me. They don't trust me. They are questioning my medical knowledge.* While a small minority of people are looking for a reason to sue (whether they have legitimate reason or not), most people just want assurance that they are making the best decision based on the most accurate information.

Research is limited, but according to one study, nearly 35 percent of second opinions are about confirming the diagnosis. More people (41 percent) want to know whether their doctor is suggesting the best treatment. Nearly 95 percent of the patients said they were satisfied with their experience of getting a second opinion, yet only 61.2 percent either agreed or strongly agreed with the second opinion. The impact of a second opinion on survival rate is extremely low. In most cases, treatment does not change. However, the data do support the value of a second or third opinion on biopsies when people receive a cancer diagnosis. The reason for this is likely that when you call for a second opinion, doctors spend more time looking through the biopsy.

Although second and even third opinions are common and expected in the medical industry, a second opinion is not sought as often as it should be because, in some cases, the outcome *does* change.

Mr. George Patel's Case

George Patel was a sixty-five-year-old public accountant who came to my office with chronic shortness of breath and an abnormal chest X-ray. His daily routine of more than ten years was to walk two miles in the morning with his wife before heading to work. One year prior to his visit, he noticed shortness of breath on exertion that gradually limited his walking distance to less than a mile. He went to see his primary doctor, who performed an extensive workup and sent him to see a cardiologist. No problems were found with his heart, but the chest X-ray showed some abnormalities, and George was referred to my clinic.

George walked into the exam room supported by his wife. He managed a few steps at a time, but even this slow pace was difficult for him. His breaths were short and labored. Darlene, my nurse, walked into my office and told me, "You need to come and see this patient now.

He doesn't look good." I ran into the room, and George was sitting up on the exam table, dripping with sweat, pale, his chest heaving with every breath.

"Hello, Mr. Patel . . ." and before I could finish my greeting, his wife interjected.

"Doctor, he can't talk. He is too short of breath, and it is getting worse by the hour. I'm scared. He is scared."

I put my hand on his shoulder, looked at his wife, and told them, "We are going to do our very best to help you. Hang in there." Within a split second, my right hand moved to his wrist to search for his pulse. It was bouncing and fast, a sign that his heart was working hard. My left hand placed a pulse oximeter on his finger, just as I was taught more than twenty years ago in medical school in Cuba. This routine is now practically part of my DNA. His O_2 saturation (oxygen level in the blood) was 81, and his heart rate an accelerated 127. His body was working hard to keep his brain and vital organs oxygenated. I called for an oxygen mask *stat*. I looked at his mouth and eye mucosa searching for signs of anemia. I then quickly performed a head, neck, chest, abdomen, and legs exam. A quick listen to his lungs revealed crackly sounds in both; it sounded just like pulling Velcro apart. George was in impending respiratory failure. We put him in a wheelchair and took him to the ER. We ordered a blood test and a CT scan of his chest. Life-threatening causes such as blood clots and heart attack were ruled out. He had no evidence of heart failure. The problem was with his lungs.

The CT scan revealed diffuse white spots in both lungs: normal lungs on a CT scan are predominantly black; his CT scan was predominantly white. It was not a bacterial pneumonia because he'd had months of progressive shortness of breath with no fever or chills. The blood test procalcitonin was normal; this helpful test excludes an active infectious process. I knew then that we were dealing with an inflammatory noninfectious process, a group of more than three hundred diseases resulting from inhalation of dust, fumes, vapors, or gases. We call them interstitial lung diseases (ILDs). A detailed history was the next step.

I interviewed his wife as if I were Sherlock Holmes, searching for all kinds of possible exposure to asbestos, toxins, vapors, and animals but could link nothing as a direct cause. This failure is not unusual. In more than 50 percent of ILD cases, we are not able to find the direct cause. The next step was to obtain a lung biopsy, a surgical procedure that requires general anesthesia. The chest surgeon uses a videoscope to access the lungs through a small hole made between the ribs. In performing this procedure, we ran the risk of not being able to remove the ventilator after surgery. At this point, a lung biopsy was essential to an accurate diagnosis. After I carefully described the risks and benefits, George and his wife agreed to the procedure.

The biopsy was performed with no complications. George was transferred to the ICU intubated on a respirator. The tissue was sent to the pathologist for analysis. The same day, I met with the pathologist who told me it would take at least a day to process and analyze the tissue. Although this time frame is not atypical, I was feeling impatient. We didn't have much time.

I went to the ICU to check on George. He was breathing comfortably on the ventilator from which he obtained 65 percent of his oxygen. Weaning off the ventilator would not be possible until the percentage of oxygen provided by the ventilator dropped below 40 percent, at which point he'd be able to breathe on his own. Finding a disease process that responds to steroids was key. If the biopsy revealed predominantly inflammation, the chances of survival increased tremendously, but if the biopsy showed fibrosis (scar tissue), a lung transplant was the only door out for George. Unfortunately, transplants are performed in select centers in the country, and intubation could disqualify George from being eligible.

The next day, I got a call from the pathologist. "Unfortunately, Gus, I cannot make any conclusive diagnosis out of this biopsy."

"What do you suggest we do?" I asked.

She shook her head and walking back to her office told me, "We need a second opinion."

"Yes, yes. But we need it *now*."

She called Dr. Armstrong, a pulmonary pathologist at a reputable clinic, who graciously agreed to review the biopsy.

"It will take forty-eight hours. You need to overnight the entire biopsy to me, and I need a day to perform the analysis," Dr. Armstrong replied.

The ICU team spent the next forty-eight hours helping George fight a good fight. Preventing complications and support was all we could do. Two days later at 9:00 a.m., I got a call from Dr. Armstrong: "Hi Gus, it is a hypersensitivity pneumonia. I made more cuts and found the classic granulomas. Is he a bird fancier?"

"No, his wife denies any exposure to birds. Thank you, thank you," I replied. I hung up the phone, ran to the ICU, put in orders for IV steroids, and gave the news to Mrs. Patel.

I started by telling her the number one thing people want to know. "It is not cancer," I said. "It is an inflammation that we can treat with steroids. Most people respond very well," I smiled. She returned the smile and folded her hands to her heart in a gesture from her native India. Bowing her head, she whispered, "Thank you."

We had a treatment, but as a scientist I was still determined to find the cause. I pushed a question I'd asked earlier related to birds: "Is there any way he would have been exposed to birds?"

"No, I told you we don't have pets, and I know no one with birds. Let me ask some of his friends."

George's response to the steroids was fantastic. Forty-eight hours after starting treatment, he was extubated and talking, able to hold a conversation. I walked into his room and joined the group of smiling nurses and family. He went on to describe how bad he had felt and how good he now felt. I was very happy for him, but deep inside I felt that my job was not finished without finding the trigger, the cause. He could be exposed again once out of the hospital and get a similar or more severe reaction.

All of a sudden I remembered reading that pillows and blankets made out of feathers have been associated with triggering bird fancier's lung, an ILD. Most people get the disease by inhaling the dust of bird droppings. It can happen to people who have birds for pets or who work in pet stores.

"Do you have a pillow or a blanket made out of feathers?"

"Yes, yes, pillows," his wife replied. "I purchased them over a year ago."

I sat down, took a deep breath in, and sighed. "That's the cause, that's the cause. We found it." I instructed his wife to remove any and all feather-based pillows from their home and to launder all bedding before George came home.

A few days later, George left the hospital walking and without oxygen. I saw him in my office a month later, and he was back to walking his two miles a day. The specialized pulmonary pathologist's second opinion made all the difference in Mr. Patel's diagnosis, treatment, and life.

In addition to potentially avoiding an unnecessary procedure or making a serious decision based on false information, second opinions can offer patients and families peace of mind. Even if the original diagnosis is found to be accurate, families usually feel some sense of relief. They've done their due diligence—they've covered the bases and haven't let important information slip through the cracks. They aren't riddled with guilt for not "doing more."

L.I.F.E.: When to Ask for a Second Opinion

Second opinions aren't always necessary, but I recommend getting one if you encounter any of the following circumstances:

L: Life-Threatening Situation. When you are in a life-threatening situation, there is usually a lot of doubt and confusion. Considering a second opinion is always helpful.

I: Intervention. When the doctor recommends a risky, experimental, toxic, or unclear treatment, make sure the team is taking the right approach. Chemotherapy, despite how common it is, is highly toxic and falls into this category.

F: Feelings. Listen to your gut and act on your feelings. If the diagnosis is not clear or if you have any doubts about the clinical team, request a second opinion. This is especially true regarding biopsies, which are misread, on average, about 15–20 percent of the time. (The percentage of misreads depends on the condition. Skin biopsies, for instance, are misread far less often than breast cancer biopsies, which have a gray zone between normal and malignant.[1]) There's a chance the pathologist is missing something in a biopsy, so I advise my patients to listen to their instincts. Your gut feeling should drive this.

E: Encouragement. A second opinion can help you calm down and feel like you have done everything for your loved one. ⤺

What Holds People Back

Most people let their initial perceptions guide their thoughts about whether a diagnosis is correct and the treatment adequate. A shiny, new, well-decorated lounge, pleasant and welcoming staff, and smiling nurses do say a lot about a facility but nothing much about the accuracy of a diagnosis and course of treatment. Doctors are only human, after all, and we have our limitations.

Another reason people shy away from a second opinion is to avoid offending the doctor. I don't usually take offense. In fact, I encourage a second opinion when I know it's important. I sometimes suggest it even when I do not believe it will change the medical outcome. For me, opening the door for patients to seek a second opinion is a way to build trust. I tell my patients, "Look, I believe that I'm doing everything that can be done on the whole planet today, in the world, but I don't have the final answer. I acknowledge that everyone has limitations, and I too have my limitations. It's possible I may have missed something, and I encourage you to get a second opinion."

By far, more people tell me, "I trust you. We are not going to go anywhere else because we are satisfied with your efforts." They have the feeling that everything has been done because I have been transparent by telling them that I am doing everything possible, but I give them permission, in a sense, to check with someone else. When I open myself up like that, when I make it clear that I will not be offended, I get incredible results. From that place of vulnerability, people sense the truth.

If your doctor does not make you feel this way, you might have to draw information out of her.

How to Approach Your Doctor for a Second Opinion

Doctors respond to reason, so I recommend using it when suggesting a second opinion. You don't need a doctor's authorization to request one, but you do want to keep your doctor informed. I recommend approaching the doctor with sincerity and reason:

> "You know what, Doctor. We think you are great, but we as a family think we are going to need another opinion. Can you suggest someone? Someone who will give us an unbiased opinion?"

> "I understand that you are busy, and I want to respect your time, but my family and I would like to know if you can refer us to someone for a second opinion. We want to have some reassurance and to know what types of options are out there for our loved one."

> This last statement is the one that the doctor is going to remember: "Listen, this is not personal, and I'm not looking to sue anyone, I just want to have answers. That's it." When you take the fear of being sued out of the picture, the oxygen in the room automatically goes up as everyone relaxes.

Be honest, be vulnerable, and be sincere. Take responsibility for your feelings. This has the effect of putting the medical team at ease. Honest, clear communication knocks down the wall physicians sometimes hide behind—the fear of being sued. When their guard is up, you are engaging in a battle. You don't need a battle. You need the truth.

❧ Google It

Online second opinions are now available from reputable hospitals such as the Mayo Clinic, Cleveland Clinic, and Johns Hopkins. You don't need a referral, to be affiliated with the hospital, or to even speak to anyone at the facility. If you aren't the patient, you will need to prove that you are the health-care agent. You will also need to upload the patient's medical records and fill out a medical questionnaire. On average, the questionnaires take about one hour to fill out. The cost for the online second opinion is usually somewhere between $500 and $800, and it is not covered by insurance. ⤞

⤐ What to Request from the Medical Records Department

Requesting medical records is a process—one almost every patient or family member needs to go through. Having copies of important medical records is necessary for second opinions. Before starting the process, make sure you know what you need. Doctors and other health-care providers are interested in seeing doctor's notes and full reports (lab, X-ray, and so on). Obtaining the records can take weeks, depending on how busy the hospital is. As soon as you know you need them, stop by or call the medical records department and request the following specific records:

- History and physical by primary physician upon admission
- Most recent laboratory reports
- Images (chest X-rays, CT scans, MRIs, and so on)—reports and images on a CD or via a link
- Medication list (active and discontinued)
- Surgeries and procedures reports (colonoscopy, endoscopy, and so on)
- Echocardiogram and electrocardiogram
- Consultants' reports (cardiologist, pulmonologist, neurologist, ICU notes)

Try to also put together a sequence of major events, as shown in the following example:

2/12/18	Admitted to the ICU
2/13/18	Intubated
2/14/18	Central line placed
3/01/18	Tracheostomy ⤞

As for My Wife . . .

Nikki is doing great. The cardiologist I initially contacted to examine Nikki is doing fine, as well. In fact, he is (and has been) a good friend of my family. He and Nikki actually work out in the same gym. But I didn't let this friendship interfere with my decision to pursue a second opinion. Nikki is far too important to me.

ACTION Practice Being Assertive

Make an effort to pay attention to how you express yourself. Some of us use the "you" word a lot: "You don't listen to me. You don't care about how stressed out I am. You never come to visit Mom in the hospital."

"You" statements tend to put people on the defensive. If you catch yourself talking that way, try to reposition the statement so that you express how you feel, rather than accuse another of doing something wrong: "Doctor, I feel unheard when you walk away as I'm speaking with you." "Doctor, I feel stressed out because I do not understand what's happening with my mom." "Sister/Brother, I feel abandoned when I am the only one at the hospital on most days." When you're assertive, you communicate a lot more—and a lot more effectively.

Caring for You

Acknowledge your emotional state. If you are having trouble staying calm, temporarily leave the room. You'll sometimes see this called "going to the balcony"—a metaphor for stepping out of the room into some actual and psychological "fresh air." By leaving the scene, you have a chance to calm down and think. You can then plan an effective response rather than react automatically.

Main Chapter Takeaways

- View the members of the medical team as your allies and treat them with respect.

- Appoint one person from your support team to be in charge of communicating with the medical team.

- Follow the communication guidelines to set a spirit of collaboration.

- Keep a list of doctors, important phone numbers, and medications.

- You deserve to be able to trust the physician in charge. If the doctor doesn't communicate well, consider approaching him or her, talking to a case manager, requesting a second opinion, or finding a new doctor.

- Consider the initialism L.I.F.E. when requesting a second opinion.

What to Do When Your Loved One Still Has Some Time

Hospice, Palliative Care, Long-Term Life Support, and Other Considerations

So far in this book, we've been talking mostly about end of life and what can happen to patients who have an advanced terminal illness that will progress despite treatment with the latest medical technology. We've covered some of the more difficult decisions and the factors that come into play when a loved one is dying in the ICU. But what happens when families or patients make the decision to employ life support? Patients on life support may live for up to a year or longer. During this time, these patients need extensive care, in the form of medication and hospital equipment as well as human touch.

Two Basic Choices

The system offers two basic choices for terminally ill patients (those with a life expectancy of six months or less): (1) LTAC with life support followed by long-term care at a skilled nursing facility with life support or (2) palliative care or hospice for those who choose to decline or to stop life support.

The goal of palliative care and hospice is to provide comfort. Palliative care can begin at diagnosis, and professionals administer or oversee most of the ongoing comfort care that patients receive. Hospice care is recommended when it is clear that the person is not going to survive the illness more than six months. Palliative care has become more accepted at any time within the process of caring for a terminally ill patient. Hospice, on the other hand, has been overshadowed by the notion that people enter hospice to die. In some ways, the hospice system is responsible for this image. Nurses don't always explain the process. Instead, they jump into talking about pain medication and morphine, positioning it as the answer to all the patient's problems.

Many of my patients reject the idea of hospice because they believe that once they sign up, morphine will be given until they stop breathing. This belief stems from a dark chapter in the history of hospice and in my opinion is the reason why the great majority of people wait until the last minute to consider it. I, for one, shared this belief about hospice for years, at least until my father-in-law was diagnosed with a terminal liver cancer and was facing the last days of his life. We brought him home from California. The first thing he told me was that he did not want needles, tubes, or cables. He wanted to die at home surrounded by family. The family met, and we all agreed to explore hospice. I was able to explain our beliefs and concerns to the hospice nurses regarding the overuse of morphine. They carefully complied with our request to administer the powerful drug only when he verbalized pain or discomfort. We—all of us, including my father-in-law—wanted some sense of control so that he would be with us, conscious, as much as possible.

Under the circumstances, it was a wonderful experience. My father-in-law was an artist, a gifted painter. During his last day on this planet, he asked us to take him outside. He wanted to see trees and flowers. The hospice team helped us, and we put him in a wheelchair. We will never forget his tremulous hands gently stretching to touch the lilies by the sidewalk. Later that day, he died peacefully, just as he wanted.

A far wider range of services is available for people who need long-term care lasting more than six months. And government resources for help are available and easy to find on the Internet. That's the good news. The bad news is that no blueprint exists for navigating today's ever-changing health-care system, and when your loved one needs long-term support, chances are you are going to face some confusion, if only because of the overwhelming amount of information you must take in and all of the factors you'll need to weigh. In this chapter, I offer you a blueprint of sorts, some immediate and ongoing goals to help you prepare for the many changes that lie ahead in terms of caregiving responsibilities, living arrangements, and insurance coverage, along with some basic information about where to turn for help.

First, let's talk about what throws people off guard from the get-go. It has to do with transition of care and is sometimes referred to as the "health-care windmill." It affects not only every patient who needs more than one level of care, but the cost of that care as well. And most people don't see it coming.

167 Days on a Windmill

After I inform patients about their clinical condition, the same questions come up in each conversation: What happens next? Where am I going to go next? What are my insurance benefits? What should I expect? One patient after another asks these questions of me every day. For most of my patients, the answer is that they will be riding the windmill of care.

Hospitals sometimes refer to the "health-care windmill" as a way to describe patient transition of care. Each vane of the windmill represents a different level of care. The move to a new vane is directed by insurance providers and the hospital—not necessarily by a doctor—which is often where the confusion begins.

The traditional windmill of health care has four vanes:

1. ICU, 7–20 days

2. Regular hospital bed, 7 days

3. LTAC facility, 25–40 days

4. Skilled nursing facility, 100 days

The exact number of days in any one facility depends on the payment arrangements the insurance company has made with the hospital. Insurance covers all or a portion of some of those stays but only for the allotted time and usually only with the insurance company's preapproval. If you'd prefer that your loved one stay in a regular hospital bed for another day or two, the doctor can request an extension, yet it's quite possible you'll be paying for it out of pocket. A fifth vane of the windmill is the trend of moving the patient home with advanced equipment. (Home health care services will most likely become a necessity as the nation's growing population of older adults overtakes hospital and nursing home beds.)

To patients and their family members, these preordained transitions of care are stressful and almost always unexpected. Families have no clue that these strict limits are in place because no one bothers to tell them until shortly before the transfer. The ICU I work in is living proof, but this pattern is not unique to my practice. These mandates, established by Medicare and followed by all health insurance companies, are nationwide. The goal is to transfer stable patients to a lower level of care where the cost is significantly less. They mean well—we need a financially sustainable system that guarantees service to all citizens. The problem I see is that the system is focused on the "money" and not on the "human being." We need a system focused on the patient without losing sight of financial stability. The only way to focus on the patients, the human beings, is to embrace them.

Lost in the System

Every day, I see people who are lost in the system. Usually, these are older adults and so-called "minorities"—a word that I don't like. I don't see people as minorities. I see people who do not understand the language or the system and who need more help than others. I see the struggles of older folks from Asian, African, European, and Hispanic communities who don't speak English. From my vantage point, I would argue that the doctors and nurses should be the leaders responsible for clear communication when it comes to next steps and transfer of care. Many of my colleagues say that they do this. However, patients and family who are experiencing a roller coaster of emotions are not always paying attention. Or they simply do not understand the language well enough. ⬎

The Numbers Speak for Themselves

My team and I surveyed families at our facility, which serves a large acute-care hospital, an LTAC facility, and two skilled nursing homes. We asked families what they knew about what was going to happen to their loved one before arriving in a hospital room. More than 90 percent of the families we talked to did not know that their loved one would be transferred from one ICU, while on a breathing machine or multiple machines, to another hospital ICU or hospital bed. Adding to the tension was that over 90 percent of the families reported that they weren't approached with the possibility of being transferred to a different location until 24–48 hours before the transfer.[1]

When family members receive news of a transfer a day or two beforehand, they often suffer the heavy psychological burden of having to watch as their loved one, attached to a breathing machine, IV, and feeding tube, is transported by an ambulance to another facility. On top of this, they have little time to research facilities or insurance benefits. ⬎

Mrs. Joan Stafford's Case

Joan Stafford, a lovely seventy-five-year-old lady who suffered a massive stroke complicated with respiratory failure that required intubation and prolonged mechanical ventilation, spent twenty days in an acute-care hospital. She did not wake up from her stroke-induced coma and was entirely dependent on the ventilator for breathing support. The decision to transfer her to an LTAC facility was made on day nineteen of her ICU stay, and her family was informed the same day. Two months later, I met Joan's daughter, Martha, in the skilled nursing home where I was seeing my ventilated patients. She told me the following story in tears:

The case manager came and told me that they found a bed for my mom at a local LTAC.

"LTAC . . . what's that?" I asked.

"Oh, I'm sorry. An LTAC is a rehab hospital for patients on ventilators. She needs it."

She told me that without hesitation. It came out of her so nonchalantly, like drinking a glass of water. I was speechless, astonished, confused, and dizzy. She offered me a tissue and a glass of water.

"Can't she get rehab here?" I asked.

"No, the LTAC is a hospital that specializes in mechanical ventilation."

"Can I go see it?"

"Sure you can. Here is the address."

"Oh no, this is forty miles from home. Is there one closer than this?"

"No, unfortunately that's the one her insurance prefers."

A few hours later, my brothers and I went to visit the LTAC. We could not believe what we saw. It was a very small hospital built in the 1950s. The lobby was the size of my bedroom closet. The hallways were clean, but the people were rude. All of a sudden, my mom went from a single bed ICU to a room shared with another patient who was also connected to a ventilator. The floor in her room had fifty years' worth of stains. The bathroom sink was from the 1960s, the air conditioning didn't work properly, and the issues went on and on. I could not believe it.

One day, the patient next to my mom seemed to be drowning on bubbling secretions, so I called out,

"NURSE, NURSE, NURSE . . . HELP . . . HELP!"

An intercom responded, "May I help you?"

"Yes, yes, the patient next to Mom is drowning on secretions!"

"Oh, okay. Don't worry. He has been like that for a year now."

I still have nightmares about this place. I wake up gasping for air and in a pool of sweat.

Forty days later, I was told that she now needs to go to another "rehab" in a skilled nursing home. Yet another lie. Dr. Ferrer, the LTAC facility had one nurse per six or seven patients. The skilled nursing facility has one per twenty. My mom's insurance covers only one place. This one is seventy-four miles away from home! I can't believe it!

Blueprint for the Transition to Long-Term Care

Knowing that the onus of communication often falls on patients and families, you should at least have some understanding of what types of questions you need to ask when your loved one is in the hospital with a terminal illness (these questions also apply to older adults who can no longer care for themselves at home and patients who are chronically ill or need rehabilitation after a stroke or a fall, for instance). Gathering this information and doing the legwork ahead of time helps you avoid being blindsided. Here is a blueprint for you to follow concerning your immediate goals:

1. Meet with your family or other support group to determine family wishes and goals of treatment. For terminally ill patients, this is unlikely to include full recovery.

2. As soon as a diagnosis has been made, ask:
   - Doctors: Prognosis and options for care
   - Hospital case manager or care coordinator: Possible locations where the patient can go and the pros and cons of each one (Keep in mind that not all facilities are created equal. A lot of them have lower standards for quality of care and focus on volume rather than the well-being of the patient.)

3. Determine what insurance will cover and get preapproval:
   - Talk to the hospital's care coordinator.
   - Call Medicare/Medicaid or your local SHIP office (see page 98).

4. Visit the facilities beforehand to see which one would be the best fit (see pages 89–90 for more detailed guidance):
   - Talk to families with personal experience at the facility.
   - Check multiple online sites for reviews.
   - Select one to three best choices.

5. Meet with family members, case managers, and doctors to establish a plan of care. This includes recommended treatments as well as recovery expectations. Bring your notes from your family meeting for goals of care (#1 above). A plan of care helps you to gauge whether the current level of care is adequate.

6. Ask the hospital for copies of specific records:
   - Medication list at discharge
   - Hospital summary highlighting procedures (dates and times) and complications

7. Schedule an interview with the care team at each of the top facilities on your list. Clearly state your goals and plan of care and ask them if they will be able to meet them. (See page 90 for specific questions to ask.)

8. Select a facility and stay aware. There's no need to be paranoid or to distrust the professionals assigned to help you and your family, but be vigilant and stay aware of what is going on with the care of your loved one.

9. Take advantage of the facilities that offer the services of care coordinators.

Getting Help from Hospital Staff

If your loved one is in a hospital setting or some level of long-term care, the staff will work with you to determine the next best level of care and then suggest some facilities, but you'll need to do the legwork and determine which one is the best fit. These days, it is more and more common for hospitals to have care coordinators on staff. So be sure to request to speak with one. Care coordinators can help in many ways. They are a liaison between you and the health-care staff, and their job spans everything from ensuring that patients understand their medical conditions to counseling patients on the different treatment options available. Care coordinators will refer you to continuing care facilities and help you get in touch with community resources. Hospital care coordinators may or may not be able to answer insurance questions, but they can lead you to the best resources.

Some long-term care insurance policies include access to a care coordinator to help with long-term care decisions. If your loved one has a long-term care policy, contact the insurer for more information. (Keep in mind who these coordinators work for. It's possible they will make recommendations that benefit the insurance company more than the patient.) Remember that the doctors and nurses who've been caring for your loved one are the most knowledgeable about his or her condition. Don't be afraid to discuss with them the care coordinator's recommendations—ask questions, run your decisions by them. These conversations can be reassuring, especially if you don't feel comfortable with all the change that's taking place.

Get the Bird's-Eye View

It's not uncommon to see chronically or critically ill patients go through a revolving door of hospitalizations, from the ICU to a hospital stay to rehab and back to the ICU. For some families, this creates a web of confusion. *Why does he have to go back to rehab? Why can't he stay in the ICU? Why didn't they just keep him in the hospital longer?* The first thing I do is sit down with them and say, "I am going to break through all those webs and try to get to what you need to know—what you need to know in terms of a thirty-thousand-foot overview of the situation." Most people don't have that. They don't have a sentence summarizing the situation. Ask your loved one's doctor to sit down with you and give you this kind of overview. ⤸

🍃 There's No Code for "Normal"

Some patients have charts with fifteen to twenty diagnoses—one for each visit. Make sure you know *the* diagnosis that is keeping your loved one in the hospital. Here's what happens: The medical insurance billing system dictates that a code be entered for each set of symptoms and resulting treatment—for example, anxiety medication prescribed for a heart patient who can't sleep. In this case, to be reimbursed for the medication and the doctor's time, the hospital must submit the "anxiety" code. This information makes its way into the medical record. This particular patient, who needed a sleep aid for just a few nights, left the hospital believing he had an anxiety disorder.

The point is that there is no diagnostic code for "normal." To be paid, hospitals must submit a diagnosis. If you're confused, talk to the doctor or care coordinator, who can hone in on the primary diagnosis. ⤸

Where Do Caregivers Go from Here?

At this juncture, everything in your world is changing. You've suddenly inherited a lot of new responsibilities. Once your loved one is set up in a facility or at home, your role as caregiver doesn't end. In fact, it might be just beginning. Caregivers often put themselves in second place. The attention is on the patient, and that can be a full-time job. Caregiver burnout is rampant, and it happens quickly.

Whether you've been caregiving for a while or are new to the role, you will benefit by having some goals of your own. I've numbered these goals to indicate some kind of order but know that they are ongoing, if only because the only thing we can really count on is change. You might find a wonderful LTAC facility for Mom and then need to move her to a skilled nursing facility down the road, or you as primary caregiver need to go back to work. The number one goal, however, remains the same: ask for help early—and over and over again as needed.

A Caregiver's Twelve Ongoing Goals

To minimize the stress and effort involved in caring for a loved one, follow these *ongoing* caregiver goals:

1. Gather one or two relatives/friends to help you right off the bat.

2. If health improves or deteriorates, determine the level of care needed (via medical staff, family doctor, or county aging unit screening).

3. Research and visit facilities, if relevant.

4. Understand insurance coverage.

5. Estimate out-of-pocket cost.

6. Discuss finances with family/lawyer and create a plan.

7. Visit patient frequently *and* take frequent breaks.

8. Be honest with yourself about how much you can handle.

9. Find ways to practice self-care: support groups, scheduled outings, walks, prayers.

10. Keep growing your support system.

11. Communicate specific needs to your support system (be nice and specific).

12. Slow down, be mindful, and keep your boundaries.

Ask for Help Early

Most caregivers wait too long to ask for help. Before they know it, they're overwhelmed and don't have the wherewithal to establish a reliable support system. So the first goal is to ask for help! One or two family members or friends are essential in the beginning. Most people, when asked respectfully, easily open their arms to the opportunity to help. If you're alone, or face obstacles with family members (which is common), support is still available to you in many forms—church, support groups, county services, and more. Talk to a nurse or doctor or care coordinator. *Someone will find someone to help you.* Overlooking this important step puts you in the position of having to make difficult life-changing decisions alone while anxious and stressed out. Knowing someone else is in your corner—and who is there to give you needed respites—goes a long way.

Determine (or Reassess) Level of Care

The options for long-term care have expanded in recent years to accommodate people who don't need a full-service skilled nursing facility but who still need some assistance. These choices are comforting to those who flat-out reject the idea of living in a nursing home, especially if all they need is a service like Meals on Wheels. Many of the options are far less costly than a nursing home as well. You'll want to gather your support group and discuss the options. You'll most definitely want to consider Mom's or Dad's wishes right up there with the doctor's prognosis. You'll be weighing many factors—medical needs, cost, location. Most families know when they've made the right decision. It won't always be ideal, but as long as the focus is on the patient, you're doing the best you can—and that's all you can do.

All levels of care require some preparation and, in some cases, a bit of training.

Mr. Frank Lee's Case

Frank Lee, a wonderful, caring husband and father of two boys, was admitted to my ICU with severe pneumonia. Now sixty-seven years old, he had smoked one to two packs of cigarettes a day for more than fifty years. Ten years ago, he began battling severe COPD, a term used to describe a hodgepodge of breathing conditions, including chronic bronchitis and emphysema, that have advanced to the point of being irreversible. COPD evolves over many years, from a noticeable but manageable shortness of breath during exertion to difficulty breathing while at rest. Coughs also tend to be progressive and disturbing.

Three or four trips to the ER per year with COPD exacerbation was part of Frank's life, his wife, Mary, told me. On this particular admission to the ICU, we intubated Frank and eventually performed a tracheostomy for prolonged ventilation. After ten days, we transferred him to a local LTAC facility, but after two weeks, he was rushed back to our hospital with a severe rectal bleed caused by a tube inserted ten days prior when he had developed liquid diarrhea.

Frank improved quickly but remained on the ventilator. With a weakened immune system, the typical complications of hospital-acquired pneumonia, skin ulcers, and urinary tract infections were just a matter of time. For Frank, every complication would be a set-back, something more to keep him from going home. We discussed going back to the LTAC facility, and he emphatically refused. He was determined to go home, and Mary agreed with his choice. They began making arrangements for at-home palliative care.

The trip home required two days of preparation. After talking to Medicare, the family was preapproved for a hospital bed, a system to suction secretions, oxygen tanks, bed supplies, medications, a nebulizer machine, two portable ventilators (one for backup), the appropriate drugs, and miscellaneous items. Medicare also approved a visiting nurse for one hour a day, Monday through Friday.

Their sons agreed to pay a nurse for a few more hours a day to give Mary a break, but they could not afford a respiratory therapist to help with the ventilator. Ventilators have a multitude of safety parameters designed to prevent a range of potential complications: if a patient receives too much air, for instance, it will blow up the lungs and create a pneumothorax (when air escapes the lungs and infiltrates the area between the lungs and the chest wall), a complication we call barotrauma. Other, simpler but no less harmful complications can take place: patients can get disconnected, the tracheostomy tube can come out, the lungs can bleed from suctioning trauma, or the tubing system can get blocked with mucus. All of the aforementioned can turn into life-threatening problems that respiratory therapists are trained to prevent and treat. Nurses are the jacks-of-all-trades. They can help with just about any aspect of home health care, but they are not schooled in working with the specifics of mechanical ventilation. Our staff respiratory therapist trained Mary on how to handle the basics of the mechanical ventilation and the necessary treatments and instructed her to call 911 if anything out of the ordinary happened. She also gave her some general precautions, such as the importance of keeping the head elevated at forty-five degrees to prevent pneumonia, and one of our nurses provided instructions on how to care for the skin to avoid wounds.

Mary felt comfortable enough with her new duties, and she seemed to comprehend how much her world was going to change because of them. Still, the preparation had just begun.

"Dr. Ferrer," Mary began, "Frank wants to spend the last days of his life overlooking the ocean. He has lived all his life in Key Largo, and our house is by the ocean. His dad built this house in 1931. It was empty back then. . . ." Her phone rang, abbreviating our conversation. It was the medical equipment company at their house. She talked to them for a few minutes. Suddenly, she changed her tone. She sounded frustrated and anxious.

"What happened?" I asked.

"I forgot to tell them that we live in a two-story house. The delivery man needs help carrying the equipment up to the second floor." She called her son, who went to help.

Five minutes later, another call. "Oh no, oh no . . . I can't believe it!"

"What happened?" I asked again.

"We can't leave today. We need to call Florida Power & Light."

"Why?"

"We don't have a backup generator. FP&L needs a letter from you explaining the need for power-outage protection in our house."

Despite these early complications, Frank left for home the next morning. A month later, my son and I visited the family, and Mr. Lee was doing great! He was now spending a few hours off the ventilator every day and relaxing on a recliner. Mary had become an expert at handling the Hoyer Lift, a hydraulic-powered contraption used to lift and transfer patients with minimal physical effort. And they were happy to be home. We talked about the transition out of the hospital. Mary kept repeating, "What a trauma, what a trauma . . . but it was worth going through it." As I write this chapter, Frank has been home for six months, on the ventilator only at night, drinking coffee in his recliner in the morning while overlooking the ocean.

Levels of Long-Term Care

Long-term care is provided in a variety of facilities. Here's a quick primer.

Long-Term Acute Care (LTAC) Facilities. These are hospitals with twenty-four-hour nursing, respiratory therapists, daily doctor visits, and rehabilitation services. Some LTACs house an ICU.

Long-Term Care Facilities. These facilities provide restorative care, skilled nursing, and other assistance for those who cannot live on their own. These include nursing homes, rehabilitation facilities, inpatient behavioral health facilities, and long-term chronic care hospitals.

Residential/Continuing Care Communities. These are apartments affiliated with long-term care facilities. They offer a range of care, from assisted living to skilled nursing, on one campus.

Adult Care Facilities. These facilities provide twenty-four-hour supervision and assistance with minimal personal care (bathing, grooming, supervision of medications, meals, housekeeping, and social activities).

Assisted Living Programs. These programs combine an adult care facility with a home health-care agency for added health-care supports, including some nursing services and doctor-ordered therapies. ⬎

Safety, Comfort, *and* Independence

Trials and tribulation are par for the course when it comes to transition of care. When it gets frustrating, remember the primary goals of any kind of long-term care: to ensure that your loved one is safe and comfortable. Most people also insist on maintaining as much independence as possible. I can't tell you how many of my patients choose freedom over safety, even those who are terminally ill. Mark, one of my patients, is a prime example.

Mark called himself a "free range" human being. He got claustrophobic when I would close the exam room door. He told me that he always kept room doors open. Freedom and independence were everything to him. At age ninety-one, he was still driving. I met Mark when he ended up in the hospital with a severe urinary tract infection. He required five days in the ICU and two days on the hospital ward. Mark was ready to be discharged, but he lived alone. He would need help getting up and moving around. Our team explained his options: he could go to an LTAC or a skilled nursing facility. "No way," he announced. Home and freedom were his only goals.

A couple of days later, we were able to discharge Mark, and he was strong enough that we acquiesced to his request to go directly home. Before discharge, we talked about safety at home and how to respond to similar events in the future. He was quick to answer. "I just want to be independent until they close my coffin. I'm DNR/DNI. If I don't get better with treatment, please just let me go. If I get better, let me be free."

Not everyone is as resilient as Mark in their nineties, and going home may not always be an option. If independence is a priority, whenever possible, start out small and add services as necessary.

When Your Loved One Is at Home

If your loved one is at home and you suspect she needs some assistance, many resources are available to you. Start out by speaking with the family doctor. Explain what changes you've noticed in her behavior. The doctor will offer advice and resources.

You can also contact your county agency on aging and disability to request a long-term care assessment. These screenings are usually free and conducted by a professional who comes to your home. They can also help to determine whether Mom is eligible for Medicaid.

By contacting these resources, you're engaging with the system, which gives you not only access to the people who have the answers to your questions but answers to questions you didn't think to ask. It's just a start, but it gets the ball rolling.

A Word to At-Home Caregivers

Communities in general are not as tightly knit as they once were. We click the garage door opener, park the car, and walk inside the house. Some of us don't even know our neighbors anymore. Just like it takes a village to raise a child, it takes a community to care for an older or ill adult. I implore you to take advantage of supports. Believe me when I tell you that most people wait too long. They believe they can handle caring for an older adult or that health will improve quickly. Many caregivers don't want to bother others or don't believe anyone will willingly chip in. They find themselves depressed and exhausted and bitter because no one will help.

In truth, it may just be that no one knows what kind of help you need exactly. From the outside looking in, it might appear as if you have everything under control. Or people don't want to meddle. And if they've never done any caregiving for an older adult before, they likely have *no comprehension* of what it involves.

So the best advice I can impart here is to convince you that *everyone* needs a support system, in the form of relatives, friends, neighbors, and in many cases personal care aides, social workers, and clergy. Once we burn out, our ability to help diminishes considerably. Then what do we do?

It's also true that not everyone is a born caregiver. We may want with all our heart to take care of Dad at home instead of placing him in a nursing home, but the planning and details and the work itself are just not natural to us. Or we're still trying to hold down a full-time job at the same time. There's no shame in this, but it is important to recognize that we're approaching a breaking point and talk about it to find a workable solution. We all have a breaking point. Staying strong is admirable, but keeping our need for help a secret can make us bitter and prone to lashing out at others. We may become the drama queen, the nightmare no one wants to help because we can't have a simple conversation without it erupting into a full-fledged knock-down, drag-out argument.

The Breaking Point

Recently, I was treating a patient with multiple medical problems. His wife, Liz, had a very pleasant nature. She was among the nicest people I'd ever met, in fact. Over the course of three weeks, her husband was transferred from one hospital to another, from rehab and back. He was eventually brought back to my hospital. By the time he got to our hospital, Liz was frustrated and angry. She called her family in for the first time, all of them. She was barking orders, admonishing them for not showing up earlier, and blaming them for how troubled she felt. When a family member tried to calm her down and ask what she needed, she produced a series of venomous responses, none of which directly answered the question.

I was shocked to see this—she had just brought these innocent family members into the picture—yet I understood. I knew her drastic change in behavior was because she hadn't been sleeping, and the transfers were unexpected and stressful. She had already spent three weeks at her husband's bedside.

Liz is a successful business woman. She runs about twenty retail stores in just as many major airports. In her business life, she knows how to take charge. Yet in her personal life, she hadn't been able to gauge when to call in the troops for help. She waited too long. When she finally rallied them, she was so mean and spiteful that no one really wanted to help.

❦ At-Home PCAs and Medicare

All or part of the cost for an at-home personal care aide (PCA) might be covered by insurance or Medicare if the patient requires some skilled nursing services, physical therapy, or speech pathology services. As of this writing, Medicare does not cover personal care, meals delivered to home, twenty-four-hour care, or housekeeping. ❧

❦ Geriatric Care Managers

Geriatric care managers (GCMs) are newcomers to the field of at-home care, and not many people know about them. Families pay out of pocket for GCM services, but a good GCM can save you money in the long run, so it's worth at least looking into the cost. GCMs are particularly valuable in helping families who are caring for someone at home and need help with caregiving *and* advocacy. They tend to have more skill sets than personal care aides because they understand the health-care system as well as insurance and resources available. GCMs can assess the level of care needed; develop a care plan; communicate with medical providers, family caregivers, and the patient; contact the right resources; decipher medical records and explain in layman's terms what is going on; and much more. I would look for a recently retired nurse or physician who might have time to do this work. A good GCM will guide, advise, and comfort the patient and family. ❧

Research and Visit Facilities

If you determine that Mom or Dad needs to stay in a facility, you'll want to investigate. Use the resources at your disposal (care coordinators, nurses, family, people you know who have loved ones in the type of facility you're looking into) to come up with a list of appropriate sites. Write them down in a notebook and leave plenty of room for comments. You'll want to do at least some of the following:

- Check the online reviews.

- Talk to your resources about what you read and get their input.

- Prepare a list of questions.

- Select the top three choices and make appointments to tour them.

- Note your first impressions:
    - Is it clean? Does it smell fresh?
    - What is overall employee morale?
    - Are patients treated respectfully?
    - Do patients seem comfortable there?
    - Are rooms cheerful and personalized?

- Interview your tour guide—or request to speak to a manager.

- Request to see an inspection report.

Questions for Long-Term Care Facilities

When visiting a facility, clearly state your goals and ask if they will be able to meet them. Ask specific questions. For instance, if a goal is rehabilitation after a stroke, your questions might include these:
- How do you define "rehabilitation"?
- How often do you perform these services?
- How often will Mom get out of bed?
- Will you teach us (family) how to help with rehabilitation?
- What is the specific plan for weaning off the ventilator?
- How often will a doctor visit Mom?

The Dark Cloud Over Nursing Homes

Of the thousands of patients I've treated over the years, not a single one has wanted to go to a nursing home, for either LTAC or long-term care. Not one. Some patients will even reach out to insurance to appeal the transfer. This "n" word is not well received by anyone needing long-term care, quite possibly because nursing homes in general have an overwhelmingly negative reputation that precedes them. Yet nursing home stays are in many cases a necessity. How do we reconcile sending our loved one to a nursing home against his or her will, especially if we can't be sure we can trust the services?

For many doctors who are in the position of recommending the transfer, this is the proverbial elephant in the room. Doctors are rooting for recovery. We want to see the disease process resolve and the patient heal. Whether that healing takes place in a regular hospital bed or a nursing home bed, however, is not up to us. We really have no control, and so we must transfer patients to the next level of care.

We've all heard stories of fraud and neglect over the years. Older adults remember when nursing homes were completely unregulated and had an even darker reputation. Some will recall the days of the almshouse—which many people knew as the poorhouse. Before the 1930s, older adults who couldn't live on their own and were isolated from family lived among the homeless and the drug addicted in an almshouse. They had a roof over their head but no medical attention. Conditions were less than desirable.

At worst, people equate nursing homes with taking advantage of the elderly. At best, they see them as cold and lonely, a far cry from home. So how much is perception and how much is fact?

These days, nursing homes are regulated more than nuclear energy facilities, yet many of them suffer from problems. As in most operations, these problems start from the top and work their way down the chain. The typical scenario involves owners focused primarily on profit and managers who are not trained in compassionate and patient-centered care. When quality of care isn't on the radar screen, we've got a recipe for disaster: the smell of urine upon entering a room, patients lying in their waste for far too long, bedsores, disgruntled employees, and high employee turnover rates. Stories of fraud and neglect in nursing homes are all over the Internet. And it's a shame.

In Cuba, I did not see such conditions. Rooms smelled fresh, and bedsores were few and far between. It is possible to care for older adults with dignity and respect. Patient-centered nursing homes exist in the United States. You just have to find them.

According to the 2010 US Census, only 3.1 percent of older adults live in skilled nursing facilities—down from 4.5 percent in 2000.[2] The remaining 96.9 percent have taken advantage of the many alternative arrangements available. If your loved one must go to a nursing home for short-term or long-term care, you will want to do your research. Not all nursing homes are created equal, so you must do some legwork and find a facility you feel comfortable with.

When Your Loved One Is in a Nursing Home

When a family member is in a nursing home, the most important thing you can do is to show up. Make regular visits and get to know the caregivers. Show up at different, unexpected times, if possible. Or have a friend or relative check in.

Ask your loved one how he feels about the place. Your loved one might have made up his mind that he didn't like the place before he even got there, but gauge his reactions to try to discern whether there's any truth to negative comments. Follow up with staff if you feel something isn't right. If you're deeply concerned, talk to the administration. If you don't find answers, report the facility to the state and do what you can to make alternate arrangements.

Check for pressure ulcers, or bedsores. Many people believe that bedsores are a given when a patient must spend months or years bedridden. But that's simply not true. Bedsores can be avoided by keeping the skin clean and dry and repositioning the patient regularly—every fifteen minutes or so for patients who can move themselves and every two hours for those who need to be moved. Nursing homes have a responsibility to prevent bedsores, yet according to the Centers for Disease Control and Prevention, an estimated 12 percent of nursing home patients develop them while in a nursing home. Bedsores are painful and, if untreated, can become infected. Malnutrition, edema (swelling), chronic vascular problems, and chronic kidney disease are among the most common predisposing factors for the development of bedsores. Although many wonderful nursing homes do a superb job in preventing and managing bedsores, others do not. Bedsores could be considered a sign of neglect, so be aware.

Having said all that, many nursing homes are stepping up. In recent years, I have worked with a growing number of nursing homes in south Florida that do a fantastic job caring for their clients. The ones that invest in staff education and facility maintenance usually do a great job. I usually recommend families do their research. Once in the facility, I suggest family members learn how to do bed rotations (repositioning the patient to prevent bedsores) and the in-bed basic physical therapy. I suggest they get involved!

Who Makes the Decision?

What do you do if your loved one refuses to go to an LTAC facility, for instance? This happens all the time, but eventually your loved one will be transferred out of the hospital. The social worker on staff plays a large role in convincing the patient and family, who are usually told that they will be responsible for paying the bills after this day if the patient stays. If you have power of attorney, you can make the decision, but you are also responsible for the bills.

Transition of care is inevitable. People do not stay in ICUs or hospital wards forever. At this juncture, many families become conflicted. They have the information, and now they must weigh all the factors, including goals of treatment, plan of care, patient's wishes, and quality of the facility or at-home care. Suddenly, finances take center stage. As a caregiver or family member, you need to protect your finances, yet you want to be sure that Mom or Dad is in a nice place. Many people struggle with this. How do we reconcile putting Mom in a

Medicaid-approved facility that we don't approve of? Do we sacrifice our financial stability? When does not contributing financially become selfish, and when does contributing become foolish?

Once a facility or at-home care is selected and the benefits have been sorted through, most families realize for the first time the significant cost involved in long-term care—in both time and money. Medicare and other insurances only cover so much, and so now families must also face another sensitive subject: the out-of-pocket cost of long-term care.

ACTION Be Proactive

As soon as caregiving is on the radar screen, call a meeting with family members for suggestions about how to handle it. Bring up roles, responsibilities, and finances. This helps ensure everyone is aware of what's needed and what's involved. Schedule regular meetings.

Caring for You

Begin or maintain a meditation practice. If you're in the thick of caregiving, find ten minutes of quiet time. The easiest way to start is to sit quietly and focus on taking deep breaths. Meditation can be more restful than sleep, so keep doing it, even if you don't feel results right away. The more you do it, the more effective it is.

Main Chapter Takeaways

- Many long-term care options exist today, making it easier to meet patient needs.

- Medicare has strict limits in place regarding how long it will pay for a patient in the hospital or long-term care facility.

- Transfer of care from a hospital bed is inevitable and a source of stress and confusion for many people.

- For a smoother transition of care, tackle the blueprint for immediate goals.

- Caregivers have ongoing goals, the most important of which is developing a support system.

- Caregivers may need to reassess level of care.

- Visit patients in long-term care facilities frequently and monitor their condition.

5

Who Pays?

Medicare, Spending Down, Long-Term Care Policies, and More

Money seems to be a cold and hard topic of conversation when it comes to life and death—another sensitive and taboo subject. Yet it's a topic most families must bring up somewhere along the care continuum because, ultimately, patients needing long-term care are faced with out-of-pocket expenses.

Long-term care is expensive—a $300 billion industry in the United States. How expensive it is for your loved one depends on the type of care needed and family circumstances. For instance, at-home hospice is typically far less expensive than a nursing home but requires that someone, whether family member, friend, or hired help, be available to tend to the patient and home when nurses, social workers, and other caregivers stop by. That cost is different for every family and includes more than money—it also includes time and energy. Is someone already at home? Does someone have to permanently give up a job or take a leave of absence? Are enough family members able to pitch in to avoid hiring a professional caregiver?

And then there's the million-dollar question: will insurance cover any or all of the services needed?

🦢 Medicare Coverage

Cost is an important factor for families when selecting a level
of care. For help in understanding what Medicare covers,
online resources are a good place to start:

- Contact your State Health Insurance Assistance Program
  (SHIP). Every state has one of these federally funded
  programs. Visit medicare.gov to find your state's SHIP
  office. SHIPs might also be able to direct you to the many
  free resources available in your county.
- Visit medicare.gov and medicaid.gov. These websites are
  designed to answer most of your general questions. 🦢

We Don't Always Have You Covered

Medicare and other insurance providers have detailed guidelines about
what is and is not covered. These guidelines seem to change rapidly
and regularly. The interesting and unfortunate part of this is that, as
health-care providers, we have limited knowledge of what happens
with those benefits. I don't blame anybody for not knowing because,
in all honesty, it would nearly take a college degree in health insurance to understand all of it. We do know that families will eventually
confront out-of-pocket spending. The gaps in Medicare coverage are
numerous and add up quickly: premiums, copayments, deductibles,
and long-term care facilities. Medicare Supplement Insurance, also
called Medigap, is designed to help older adults avoid being nick-
eled and dimed to bankruptcy. Medigap helps cover copayments and
deductibles, but it doesn't cover special diets, medical equipment,
home health care, or health care when traveling out of the country.

Many, if not most, of my patients and their families are surprised
to learn what is not covered. Fear consumes them as they realize the
number of losses they are facing: the health of a loved one, the possibility of having to put him or her in a facility that is affordable but not
high quality, and financial stability. How much can a nursing home
take from a patient or spouse? How do loved ones reconcile whether
to help pay for care?

Mrs. Hilda Swenson's Case

Hilda Swenson was an eighty-two-year-old widow when I met her in a skilled nursing home. Three months prior she had suffered a stroke that left her unconscious and attached to a ventilator for breathing support. She had been a teacher for four decades, and she had handled her finances very well. Her home was paid off, and she had saved a small fortune, but she was using more and more of her retirement funds to cover medications, physical therapy, and doctor's visit copayments. Hilda didn't have any children. Marilyn, her seventy-seven-year-old sister, and Nancy, her niece, were Hilda's primary caregivers.

Hilda never regained consciousness, and she required the ventilator for breathing support. By the time I met Hilda, she had twenty-five days left of the Medicare coverage allowed for long-term care, a detail that the skilled nursing facility's business office communicated to Marilyn and Nancy. The two women were shocked to learn that Medicare limits the number of days it will pay for a nursing home stay. Even worse, they learned that they—the patient and her family—were responsible for the bill beyond the one hundred days allowed by Medicare. Because Hilda had some financial resources (a home and a bank account), she was not eligible for Medicaid.

Once Medicare coverage for the skilled nursing home ended, Marilyn and Nancy tapped into Hilda's finances to pay the daily $500-plus they had agreed to pay the facility. Forty days later, they ran out of money, so they quickly sold Hilda's house and jewelry and used the money to pay the bills. Five months later, Hilda was "chronically stable," evolving from one complication to another—pneumonia, urinary tract infections, and diarrhea—but nothing major. When Hilda's money ran out, Marilyn and Nancy began to use their own. Finally, they contacted a lawyer who helped them apply for Medicaid on Hilda's behalf. This time, she was eligible—their financial ruin qualified Hilda for government help.

Typical Out-of-Pocket Health-Care Costs at the End of Life

In 1990, the National Institute on Aging and the Social Security Administration began sponsoring the Health and Retirement Study (HRS), a longitudinal study on health, retirement, and aging. The goal was to collect data on how our changing world affects the well-being of adults aged fifty and older. This data includes information obtained from "exit interviews," or conversations with a family member of a recently deceased survey participant. Researchers can then use this data to conduct studies. When it comes to financing end-of-life care, several studies look at Medicare expenditures. Few studies, however, look at out-of-pocket costs.

Using HRS data from the state of Michigan, researchers looked at lifetime health-care expenditures and determined that, per capita, the average cost is $316,600, nearly half of which is spent during the senior years.[1] Different researchers looked at average out-of-pocket health-care expenditures for older adults, with a special focus on end-of-life expenditures. As it turns out, Medicare, as much of a blessing as it is to Americans aged 65 and older, only scratches the surface of some of the financial burden, especially during the last year of life. So who foots the bill?

End-of-Life Out-of-Pocket Health-Care Expenditures

As of this writing, in 2017, the average "nonhousing" wealth of a typical retired older adult in the United States is $25,000. Last-year-of-life care expenditures total, on average, about $12,000 for nursing home and hospital care, insurance, prescription drugs, home health care and helpers, and spending to make the home accessible. But people can—and do—spend a lot more.[2] According to a MetLife survey, the average cost of a private room in a skilled nursing facility in 2012 was $248 per day, or $90,520 annually. Some people who can afford it opt to spend up to $75,000 per month. Assisted living runs about $118 per day. Home health aides charge about $21 an hour.[3] Cost varies based on the type of facility and location. You might pay much more in Alaska, for instance, than in Oklahoma.

It's hard to quantify long-term care expenses. Most of the research is based on hospital stays. And cost varies from state to state and depends on the types of services needed and for how long. But no matter how you slice it, long-term care is expensive relative to the wealth of the average person.

The Bigger Questions

How do we understand our options in this day and age when people are living longer and on limited incomes? How do we settle recurring copays and hefty deductibles? Does the size of a bank account determine how long a patient lives or the quality of care he receives? Are family members compelled to empty their coffers to care for an aging parent with no funds of his own? Are spouses expected to remortgage or sell their home and deplete retirement savings? How are they to survive? How do families manage this financial burden? These questions take on increasing importance, given that we are, as a rule, living longer.

Most of Us Will See Some Gray

Until fairly recently, few people had to think about preparing for old age. It wasn't an issue because most people didn't live past the age of sixty-five or seventy. Life expectancy occasionally drops in the United States, but for the most part it has steadily increased. We're living long lives here in the United States, where the average age of death for men is 76.3 and for women it's 81.2, which means that, with increasing regularity, many of us are living into our nineties. According to the US Census Bureau, the number of Americans eighty-five and older is expected to increase from 5.9 million in 2012 to 8.9 million by 2030—and to a staggering 18 million by 2050.[4]

To get a stronger picture of how these numbers compare to life expectancy for earlier generations, let's look at how significantly these numbers have changed over the past century. In 1900, life expectancy for men was 46.3 and for women 48.3. In 1918, at the start of the United States' entry into World War I and the worst flu pandemic in recorded history, it dropped by ten years—36.6 and 42.2. By the mid-twentieth century, life expectancy had risen, nearly doubling to 65.6 for men and 71.1 for women.[5]

Now that medicine has helped extend the average life expectancy by about thirty years since the beginning of the twentieth century, millions of people are living to an age when health naturally begins to deteriorate. Add to that the size of the population entering their senior years, and we have the potential for a record number of Americans relying on the health-care system for everything ranging from routine doctor visits to taking up residence in a nursing home. And not many of us are prepared for this—neither individuals, families, the government, nor the health-care system.

Rising health-care costs and limited retirement savings, combined with Social Security benefits we can't be certain will be available in years to come as well as longer life expectancy, spell financial strain for most families. Given these facts, we can safely predict that most of the population will need to make some important and difficult financial decisions about how to care for a chronically or terminally ill relative in what is likely to be an underfunded and overcrowded health-care system for those who need long-term care. I've seen many families suffer devastating financial hardship in an effort to finance their own care or that of a spouse or other loved one. Medicaid is there to help, but only after most assets have been exhausted.

Spending Down

To pay for long-term care services, patients are expected to "spend down," or use their assets to cover the costs. Most patients begin by digging into personal funds, including Social Security checks, savings, pensions, IRAs, stocks and bonds. Some people have long-term care insurance (LTCI), a more recent phenomenon. LTCI covers some long-term care expenses for people who want to protect their assets and avoid spending down. And people who have a life insurance policy with an accelerated death benefit rider might be eligible to receive a portion of the insurance paid to them under certain circumstances.

Once liquid assets are exhausted, material assets come into play. Some people take out a reverse mortgage on their home. Others sell homes, cars, and other valuables. The rules for spending down vary by state, and some assets are protected.

Financial loss puts families and patients in a great deal of turmoil. In some cases, it becomes a major distraction.

Ms. Hermosa Acosta's Case

Hermosa loved her job as a part-time cashier in Sedano's, a Cuban grocery store in Miami. She lived in a modest home in a Miami suburb, where she had resided for most of her life after emigrating from Cuba in 1950. She was thirteen years old when her father brought her family to Tampa on a business trip. She fell in love with Tampa and asked her dad to allow her to study in America. They stayed, and seven years later, Hermosa met her husband in Tampa. Eventually, the couple moved to Miami to work for Sedano's. Hermosa's husband was a manager who regularly worked overtime to enable them to purchase a house. At the age of seventy-five, her husband passed away of a heart attack. Two years later, Hermosa found herself suffering from ill health.

In her mid-seventies, Hermosa was diagnosed with uterine cancer and underwent surgery that resulted in a complication. She bled into her chest cavity and landed in the ICU hours later, where I ordered that she be intubated and attached to a breathing machine. After ten to fifteen days in the ICU, she required a tracheostomy. A longtime smoker, she had some lung issues to begin with. Although we were able to eventually remove the respirator, she suffered from many respiratory problems and remained unconscious for the duration of her stay in the ICU.

Hermosa's only living family consisted of a distant nephew. She had planned to help the nephew when she died by leaving him her house, savings, and belongings, yet she was unaware that he had moved back to Cuba. Eventually, Hermosa was transferred to an LTAC facility, where she stayed for a couple of months, and during that time she regained consciousness. We placed a speaking valve (called a Passy-Muir valve)—a one-inch cylinder with a one-way valve connected to the tracheostomy tube that was placed surgically in her neck right below the Adam's apple. The valve allows air to move through the vocal cords, so people with a tracheostomy can talk. She was pleased to hear her distorted, whispered voice for the first time after weeks on the ventilator. But instead of talking about how grateful she was to be alive or expressing some last wishes, her concern the whole time was about her house, her possessions inside the house, and the fact that she didn't have her finances in order. Her house was almost paid for, but here she was in LTAC with no family to help her take care of life's daily affairs on the outside. This troubled Hermosa to the point where she couldn't think about anything else.

Months later, I saw Hermosa again in a skilled nursing facility. She was still conscious but by then had defaulted in the payment of her property taxes. Her savings account was depleted, and the bank was sending her notices about foreclosing on the home she had lived in for nearly thirty years. She didn't have family or anyone who could have helped her rent or sell the house. Hermosa was deeply distraught. And she could do nothing to satisfy her nagging desire to get out of the hospital and go back home to try to put things in order. Above all, she could not contact the only living relative that she had. Hermosa was basically swallowed up by the system because she didn't know how to defend herself or protect herself in this situation. And no one, including hospital staff, seemed to be able to help.

In just four short months after getting ill, Hermosa lost a lifetime of savings and was on the verge of losing all her possessions.

She died in the nursing home about seven months after leaving the ICU; she spent the last three months of her life impoverished.

Hermosa's story is not unusual. Although most people have a friend or family member to help at the end of life, many people need long-term care long enough to deplete their assets, or what they thought would be their family's inheritance.

Even those who saved well for their retirement are living long enough to deplete their assets, and many more rely on Social Security and Medicare or Medicaid to pay for doctor visits, tests, surgeries, rehabilitations, and long-term care facilities. An increasing number of older adults and chronically ill people need help that goes well beyond asking or paying someone to do light housework and run errands. These people enter a health-care system that, although technologically advanced, isn't necessarily designed to fully finance long-term care for everyone. And as rewarding as caring for an older adult can be, it's neither glamorous nor well paying. Many long-term facilities are over-crowded and must contend with high staff turnover, which leads to families questioning the quality of care being offered.

Most of us are at least vaguely aware of these facts. And we might know some details about Mom's coverage—that she has Original Medicare with prescription drug coverage (Part D), for example. But it's likely we haven't studied the policy. Rather, we assume Medicare or Medicaid will cover the essentials. I find over and over again that most families and patients are unaware of the limits Medicare has in place. Sometimes, it's best to turn to an expert for help.

Use Legal Resources to Create a Plan

Most families I see are so caught up in the responsibilities before them that they wing it when it comes to finances. It starts the moment a loved one ends up in the ICU. A daughter uses up all her paid time off (PTO, the term used to describe a combination of vacation, sick, and personal days) within the first week and then is at a loss when she needs to take more time off. I write letters to employers regularly, explaining that so-and-so needs time away from her job to care for her ill father. Some employers are gracious and allow employees to keep their health insurance while away from work for an extended period. Others, not so much. For most people, protecting job security is para-mount. Yet they fail to make some kind of plan.

My advice to you regarding finances is similar to my advice to you for support: make it a priority. Bring the subject up early and often and get help. This might start with your job security. Communicate with employers, know what you can expect, and make a bedside vigil sched-ule for each family member so that no one has to lose a job because someone got ill. Ask the doctor to write a letter to your employer—it makes a difference, and doctors are used to doing it. Make sure other family members are taking the same steps. At some point in time, every family suffers a crisis. Employers are also used to this.

If it's looking like long-term care is a possibility, your financial plan might have to go as deep as allocating which of Mom's assets to spend down first. Whenever possible, hire a lawyer (not a financial planner) to help you get paperwork in order and understand the rules and regulations of spending down in your state. You also want to avoid making mistakes—such as transferring money from Mom's account into yours so that Medicaid won't find it. Medicaid will find it, and you'll likely be required to pay it back at some point down the road.

Lawyers can also help Mom shelter as many assets as possible. For instance, if Mom has an IRA and has not designated anyone as heir, when she passes, Medicaid might be able to use that money to cover the cost of a nursing home. A home that has been paid off and does not have a quitclaim deed signing it over to the intended heirs can get caught up in probate court, which costs time and money. I'm not advocating for ways to "beat the system." I am encouraging you to be fiscally responsible when it comes to protecting assets your loved one worked hard for so that all is not lost. Families who hire a lawyer and come up with a viable financial plan tell me it was the best thing they could have done. They don't regret the cost. They firmly believe that they couldn't afford not to hire a lawyer.

ACTION Rely on Word of Mouth

Talk to others you know who have parents in nursing homes or other facilities. Word-of-mouth referrals can be some of the best if you trust your sources.

Caring for You

Take a few moments and give yourself permission to feel good. Treat yourself to something special. Between visits to facilities, stop for your favorite latte or ice cream—or a healthy meal.

Main Chapter Takeaways

- Long-term care is expensive, and Medicare coverage is complicated and finite.

- Half of lifetime health-care expenditures are typically spent in the last year of life.

- Americans are living long enough to exhaust their retirement savings.

- Long-term care patients must "spend down" and liquidate assets to pay for long-term care services before qualifying for Medicaid.

- Each state has its own laws regarding "spending down."

- Consulting a lawyer and creating a financial plan for long-term care is a priority.

Legacies and Regrets

The Importance of Having Final Conversations about Life

Alfred had been a heavy smoker for the majority of his seventy-four years. He was also a self-described alcoholic who hadn't been able to hold down a job for more than a couple of months at a time. A mechanic by trade, he'd sober up, find work, start drinking to excess again, and lose his employment. This pattern was the most predictable part of Alfred's life, given that he was also homeless and had been for twenty years.

The day Alfred showed up on my ward, he was suffering from severe pneumonia. The police had found him outside a gas station just two blocks from the hospital. He was flat on his back, his head resting on a pool of vomit, his right hand clinging to a can of beer wrapped in a brown paper bag. He was alone in the ER wearing ragged, disheveled clothing. If he had family and friends, he didn't let on. I wasn't convinced Alfred would walk out of the hospital. It was likely, I thought, that we strangers would be the last people he would ever have contact with.

Dying of pneumonia is not uncommon, especially when the body's defenses are low. Pneumonia is an inflammation of the lung tissue. The main windpipe branches out into smaller and smaller microscopic tubes that end up in tiny air sacs called alveoli. It's there where oxygen is absorbed into the bloodstream. The alveoli contain a thin layer of fluids, proteins, and fighting cells that clean and protect the lungs from invaders. Cancer, smoking, chemotherapy, rheumatoid arthritis, and many other chronic debilitating diseases usually impair the many biochemical pathways responsible for maintaining the integrity of the immune system—they lower our defenses. It's there where the backup system to the fighting cells in the alveoli fails. Bacteria, viruses, fungi, and foreign substances such as vomit win the battle. The body responds with alveoli filled with fluid, impairing the ability to breathe and turning mucus production from gray to yellow and then green. Each year, millions of Americans develop pneumonia, frequently as a complication from another illness, and about sixty thousand die from it. Most patients died of pneumonia prior to the ICU and antibiotics era. Sir William Osler, often described as the father of modern medicine, famously called pneumonia "friend of the aged" because it was seen as a quick, relatively painless way to die.[1]

It was obvious that Alfred's case was severe. Both of his lungs were burned by the vomit he had nearly asphyxiated himself with, creating an opportunity for common bacteria from his mouth to get into the lungs. They traveled with the vomit down to the deepest part of both of his lungs and quickly multiplied, producing a large amount of mucus—the inflammatory response. His years of smoking had destroyed most of his alveoli and the lungs' defense mechanism. Debilitated from alcohol and with a weak cough, he was drowning in his own secretions. I could hear the crackly sound coming from his chest even when standing at the door of his room. He was in obvious discomfort. I could tell by the muffled sounds of moaning coming through his oxygen mask.

When I walked in to examine Alfred, I could have given him the drill about vices. He had two of the most deadly ones, after all, both of which had consumed his health. But the futility of that was apparent—not because he was addicted (everyone is a candidate for recovery) or because I thought he was dying, but because it wasn't what he needed. He didn't need me to hammer him down even more by telling him everything he'd done wrong. What Alfred needed first and foremost was medical attention. But Alfred also needed something else. He needed someone to talk to, a conversation and a pair of ears to hear what might be his last words, his last thoughts, his regrets. He needed to be "seen," to have a witness to his life, to know he belonged, and to release some of his mental burden.

"I think you have a bad case of pneumonia, but you are getting good antibiotics and treatment, and we are going to help you," I said. "What are you going to do when you get out of here?" I didn't want to tell him about my first impression, about my sense that he would die from his pneumonia. It was too early in his hospital stay. I could be wrong, after all. At this point in my career, I knew enough to know when to hold my peace.

"Oh, I'm going to go back to the streets."

"But you are going to catch something else down the road," I explained. I had never met Alfred before, but based on the number of ER encounters listed in his medical records, we estimated that he'd been in the ER at least forty times over the past six years. He mentioned his alcoholism, and so I delved a little deeper. "Do you think that pulling out of this area where all your drinking buddies are could be a good idea?" My goal was to present some alternatives and to get him to comprehend what would happen if he continued doing what he was doing.

Our conversation got serious. "Life has limits, and it will end one day," I said. "If you keep coming to the hospital like this, and you haven't reached out to a friend or family, who is going to make decisions for you? You know, if you continue like this, and if you become unconscious, the state will decide what happens to you. You will have no control."

Aggressive treatment that included antibiotics, fluids, nebulization, and close nursing care helped pull Alfred through. By day two I found him sitting up holding a full conversation with his nurse while devouring breakfast. The crackly sound from his chest was no longer audible.

After about three days, Alfred was searching for me in the hallways. We had developed a friendship based on the most basic of human needs—to connect with others. This need is magnified toward the end of life—so much so that some people will hold on to life well beyond a doctor's estimate in order to speak their piece to one person or another.

The topics of the conversations Alfred and I had weren't necessarily uplifting, but the experience was. Alfred had shared with me some of his regrets. He told me about his upbringing in a family of alcoholics. He was eleven when his dad gave him his first hard drink; he recalled his disgust vividly. Many more came after that one—some given by Dad, uncles, and cousins, and some stolen. Soon afterward, he discovered cigarettes at school. "I tried weed and cocaine but didn't like them," he told me.

"Did you ever try injectable drugs?" I asked.

"No way, Doc. It hurts. I'm afraid of needles," he said as he giggled.

"How about your family. Are they local?"

"Doc, all of them are gone," he replied looking down and toward the window on his left. He sighed deeply, and a tear came from his right eye. I paused for a few seconds. All my questions came to a halt. I thought about my family back home in Cuba. I hadn't seen them in more than a decade. They were out of sight but not gone. I knew most of them were still alive. I even knew that if I needed them or they needed me, they were just a phone call away. In fifteen seconds I thought about all the birthdays, surgeries, hospitalizations, and deaths I had missed. Suddenly our eyes met, and he continued.

Alfred talked about the importance of family, of taking care of them. He clearly regretted that he no longer had family members in his life. For the first time, I felt how truly lonely he was. I encouraged Alfred to find an Alcoholics Anonymous group or a church—a place with people he could try to build a relationship with. I wasn't convinced he would do it, but I held out some hope that he would.

Ten days later, Alfred was discharged, and I never saw him again. One thing I know for sure is that our conversations were at least as powerful as any antibiotic. I believe they were the best medicine for Alfred.

The Healing Effect

Most dying patients want to say something before they pass. I believe it's because conversations heal. Maybe not always a complete physical recovery, like in Alfred's case, but they can do a lot to remedy the effects of pent-up resentments and regrets. Unspoken words eat away at us, but sharing them somehow makes them lose their power over us. And when we forget about the need to be right, when we can forgive and forget for the sake of forgiveness, a healing takes place that is hard to describe. Sometimes the healing is mental. Other times, it is spiritual. In cases like Alfred's, the healing manifests as physical. That is how powerful conversation can be. And so I am an advocate for conversation—not just the conversations about preparing for death that we talk about elsewhere in this book, but the ones about life. Toward the end of life, when so much of the conversation is about medical options, conversations about life are often overlooked, even avoided. But they couldn't be more important. Patients who are conscious and capable of talking have an irrepressible desire to express their thoughts.[2] In my practice, this is a recurring theme.

Mostly, people who are on their deathbed want to shed the regrets they harbor and impart some wisdom to those they will be leaving behind. Sharing is paramount in the end. It's as if people need to release their pressing thoughts, so they can leave this world with a clean slate. At the end of life, this conversation can't be postponed, a fact the dying patient is well aware of.

In many cases, the conversation starts when a dying patient willingly speaks up. Lydia was one such patient. When I removed the tracheostomy tube from Lydia's throat, she hadn't been able to speak for three months. Clearly she'd had plenty of time to think. As I sat at her bedside listening as she finally found her voice again, she told me about her life. Her biggest regret, she said, was that she'd never had any children. Then she grabbed my hand and pulled me close. "I see you working so hard," she told me. "That's good, but this is the time to be building memories with your family."

I've never forgotten this conversation because it's such a profound example of what I hear from my patients as they approach the end. Their concerns are rarely for what lies beyond. Their thoughts are often a backward glance at what once was and what could have been, and frequently they are focused on those they are leaving behind.

When the patient doesn't begin the conversation, it's usually up to a family member to start talking. Yet rarely do I see this happen. If these conversations are so important, why do we avoid them at the risk of never having them? Why are they so hard?

Last conversations about the experiences of life with someone who is dying are a source of emotional resistance. Loved ones are scared they won't find the right words or that they'll sound clichéd or inauthentic. Sometimes they are afraid of hearing or having to admit to a truth or are reluctant to give up a resentment. They get ahead of themselves and judge their behavior before they even make a move. But the bedside vigil is an unparalleled opportunity to have some of the most important conversations of life; it's something people probably don't think much about until they're faced with it. I've observed the intensity and discomfort people feel as they speak, perhaps for the last time, to a loved one. But when they break through their resistance and do it as best as they can, it produces nothing short of a miraculous healing—for everyone involved.

But what, exactly, do we say to the person who is dying? What do we say to others? What do we say to *ourselves*? The most powerful place to begin is by reassuring our loved one that we are with him.

The Power of Reassurance

Toward the end of life, people are ready to confess. They are waiting for the right time and the right person to cross their path. It could be a friend, doctor, nurse, or a family member. I believe that under the stress of illness, it is hard for people to open up and start the conversation. They need a compassionate human being who can hold their hand and help them open up their heart, someone to break the ice. They don't need instructions: "You know you are sick? Do you want to talk?" No, please, they don't need to be asked questions. Reassurance is what they need first. They want to hear, "I want you to know that I'll be here no matter what. We are going to face this together." They almost always require that someone give them a glimpse of hope. No matter how old or sick people are, they long to hear words like, "Everything is going to be okay."

Ms. Ruth Goldstein's Case

Ruth Goldstein was a seventy-nine-year-old woman with severe emphysema—a progressive disease caused by smoking. It eats up the lungs so that they resemble the appearance of Swiss cheese. She was told that she had emphysema years ago, but she never sought medical attention, something that could have helped her live longer. She considered her persistent cough and shortness of breath part of getting older. Ruth had worked as an executive in the fashion industry for forty years. She traveled much and smoked a lot. The day I met Ruth in the ICU, she had been on her way home from Europe. In New York's LaGuardia Airport she had developed a fever and chills. This strong woman pushed through half of her connecting flight before she finally decided to reach out for help, but by then she couldn't talk. Instead, wheezing sounds came from her chest. Sweaty, cold, and clammy, Ruth finally managed to mutter, "Help . . . help . . . help . . . me," with her eyes wide open and neck muscles as tight as cables holding up a bridge—a sign that someone is struggling to breathe. Her seatmate quickly summoned the flight attendant, who pulled the oxygen mask down from underneath the overhead compartment. Her breathing settled gradually. The pilot called for an emergency landing in Fort Lauderdale, the closest airport. The ambulance was there when they landed, and in less than ten minutes she was in Aventura Hospital's emergency room. Dr. Todd had been briefed by the ambulance tech, "Seventy-nine-year-old female with unknown past medical history . . . ," and he quickly mobilized the troops. Two doctors and three nurses met her at the ambulance, pulled her out, and rushed her into a room.

"BiPAP 12/5."

"Get an 18-gauge IV."

"Albuterol nebulizations."

"Lasix 40 milligrams IV and Solu-Medrol 120 milligrams IV. *Now!*"

A mask covered her mouth and nose in a tight seal. It was connected to the respirator (BiPAP) through a snorkel-like tube. One hour later, she was transferred to the ICU where I met her. By then, she was able to talk. I removed the mask, held her hand, made eye contact, and introduced myself. I told her, "You are getting better. I heard the story. I'm going to do my best to get you out of here. Is there anybody I can call for you?"

She broke into tears. I waited for a few seconds before continuing, "Listen, you are getting better, you are breathing better, and you can talk in full sentences. I need you strong. I'll help you fight through this." Then I added, "What are you going to do when you get out of here?"

She smiled and wiped her tears from her cheeks. "I thought it was over, up there in the air. No words came out when I tried to speak. 'Stay with me' was all I heard over and over. I felt some relief when we landed, but then I felt anxious and frightened by the loud sirens and the red and blue flashing lights. Then the questions started: *What's your name? How old are you? Any medical problems?* I felt as if I were being interrogated for a crime . . . almost guilty for being there. I was scared, and not one word of reassurance was spoken, not one kind word. I know they meant well and did a great job, but where was the heart, the compassion?

"Doctor, throughout my ordeal, I longed for somebody to hold my hand and tell me that it's going to be okay." She paused again, squeezed my hand, looked up at me with grateful eyes, and said, "Thank you. Your reassurance has made me feel so much better. I feel better. Thank you."

Over the course of the day, we tried removing Ruth's BiPAP. But every time she spent an hour off the BiPAP, her breathing became labored, shallower and shallower. Her husband and sons were now at her side, and they listened intently as her sentences were reduced to one-word commands: "Gary . . . ," few breaths in, "call . . . the lawyer."

"Okay, Honey, I will. Let's get you back on the snorkel mask." They both giggled. "You'll be better by the time he comes. Just take a nap."

By the next day, Ruth's ICU room had become an office. Two laptops, one connected to a portable monitor, a mouse, two yellow notepads, and several pencils covered the patient table across her bed. Ruth was striving to get her affairs in order. By now, Ruth was spending a good two or three hours off the BiPAP but quickly tired out, requiring that she be placed back on the machine. On several occasions, she came close to being intubated. However, she had made herself DNI. The idea of putting a thick plastic tube through her mouth into her lungs terrified her.

"Dr. Ferrer, if I were younger, with healthier lungs, I'd bear anything to remain alive," she had told me earlier in the day. She understood that the emphysema had eaten up her lungs and that her chances of coming off the respirator were slim to none. She knew that after a week or so with the tube through her mouth, a more permanent tube would be inserted through her neck, a surgical procedure that she did not want. "Most of the people with lungs like mine spend the rest of their days connected to machines, abandoned to rot in a nursing home. I don't want that. I want to die at home."

During my rounds the next day, I found her sitting up in bed and off the BiPAP. She smiled when I walked in. "I was able . . . to put . . . some stuff in order. The important ones . . . you know . . . house, bank."

"Is there anything we can do for you today?" I asked.

"Help me . . . go home . . . with hos . . . hospice."

I asked her to give us more time to help in her recovery. I told her that it would take more than just two or three days, but she was determined to go home.

"I won't be able to do what I want to do in the hospital," she argued. But she agreed to stay a few more days while we arranged for hospice. She gradually improved to the point that she was off the BiPAP for up to five hours. Her husband and sons were at peace with her wishes. They, too, understood that her disease was fatal. The best way they could help her now was to accommodate her wishes, not fight them. This became their way of reassuring her that they were with her, all the way.

Regrets, Wishes, and Wisdom

Once patients feel reassured, they are more likely to begin the conversation about life. During this event, these last conversations, patients are coming to terms with their life, family, job, and friends. If you think about it, this is powerful stuff. Regrets are usually the main thing that they ponder. Next is the desire to share some of their wishes, values, and wisdom with family members. As a loved one, you have the honor of being fully present and listening to what are often profound and always memorable confessions and wishes.

Do you know what the number one regret is for most people? You guessed it if you said something to do with relationships. The most common regret I have come across is "time wasted away from friends and family." Nothing can fill this longing to go back in time and create more intimacy with loved ones. Spending more quality time with children or mending a broken relationship would have remedied these feelings, but we don't realize this until we look back, and now these feelings linger, and we feel helpless to make a difference.

The second most common regret might surprise you. It is not having followed a calling—not having pursued a career or business idea. This kind of regret usually comes down to "fear of failure." I often hear, "I wonder where I would be if I had had the courage to do . . . or the guts to persist with . . ." I have seen this over and over again. I find it incredibly intriguing that, across the board, people experience the same types of regrets.

At this point, the antidote is to express the regret in the presence of someone. In some cases, family members can also create opportunities to mediate the situation. It begins with getting creative in overcoming some of our fears about communicating with a dying loved one.

Express Your Feelings:
Healing Is Always Possible

It is not difficult for people to say, "I'm sorry," or express some type of sadness when a loved one is dying. But overcoming the fear of saying what you feel deep down about a dying loved one is terrifying for some people. When I see this fear and regret, I tell family members that it's possible to do something to remedy the situation. Most people don't think this could possibly happen, but when I ask them if they would be able to write a letter or make a video or do something to express their feelings without having to come straight out and say them, they light up. It becomes instantly doable to help clear up bad feelings and regrets over whatever happened in the past.

A few years ago, Arthur, a seventy-three-year-old cancer patient, entered the hospital for what was clearly the last time. His health was failing fast. He was constantly surrounded by family members who would come two or three at a time, sitting beside his bed for hours, just staring at him without speaking. The fear and grief in the room was palpable for all, including the patient. We had to change the dynamic.

I called Devon, one of his adult children, out of the room and told him to go home and bring back some family photo albums. Soon, I began hearing laughter as they looked through the pictures. Although Arthur was no longer conscious by this point, I felt in my soul that it was a great comfort to hear his loved ones reminiscing about the good times. Devon later told me that the experience brought the family closer together and that they were finally able to talk honestly about losing someone close.

I have seen families using the time they have with the patient to express love. Some families create a diary or a journal of their time in the hospital. Instead of writing about their concerns or complaints, they somehow use the medium to express love. They do this by recording their last visits together—writing about a visitor, a treasured poem, beautiful memories, or beautiful thoughts about the person they are about to lose. I have read probably four or five diaries and journals that people have created while in the hospital, and they are entirely focused on expressing love or forgiveness or something else positive. It really is incredible how something so simple can foster so much joy.

Encouraging the Conversation

I'm not a psychologist and would never claim to know the intricacies of what it takes for a person to heal mentally and emotionally. I only know what I see—and that is that people who are conscious and able to speak harbor a pressing desire to share some thoughts before they pass. Many, however, don't get the opportunity. In a hospital setting, where clinicians are focused on whether to initiate DNR orders and where families are often confused and full of anxiety, little attention is paid to the dying patient's real need: to talk about regrets and pass on important values, hopes, and wisdom to children or grandchildren.

I see this every day. If the clinician doesn't assume this role of encouraging this communication, it likely will not happen, as patients get caught up in a flurry of activity. And so I make a point to foster these conversations between patient and clinician or patient and loved one.

Wisdom and Values

Dying patients usually tell you something that is not related to their disease process or today's issues. Although they want to be informed about their condition, their main worry is about family and expressing love and forgiveness and passing on some wisdom. Alongside—or in place of—regrets is the deep desire to impart wisdom and values to family members.

I took care of a young lawyer. She was fifty-two years old and dying of lung cancer, even though she had never smoked. When she arrived in the ICU, she was able to speak and express her wish not to be treated. What happened while caring for her in the weeks afterward became another one of those life-changing experiences for me. I walked into her room one morning before rounds. She was short of breath and wearing an oxygen mask. I acknowledged her husband and then asked her if there was anything I could do for her that morning, and she told me no, with a nod of her head. I then added that I wanted to talk to her about what was in her heart. "You don't want to miss this opportunity to talk, to express what is in your heart. You are still conscious and here with us." I held out one of those writing pads that we give patients. She was always writing things down because she couldn't talk due to the mask. I stood next to her as she used her shaky hands to write on the pad. The first thing she wrote was "kids." She had three kids, and so her husband and I began asking questions, trying to discover what it was exactly that she wanted to communicate about her children. For every question we asked, she would nod yes or no. After an hour of going back and forth with her scribbles and trying to interpret what was on her mind, we realized that it was all about what she wanted to tell those kids before she left this world. She wanted to talk about her dreams for them. Her husband knew her so well that he was able to come up with the things that she wanted to say. It was about her home and her relationships and about following the values that she follows and to wait for dating until they finish high school. We deciphered all of that through her shaky handwriting. She wanted to express all of this, but if the conversation had not been initiated, it might not have happened. Twenty-four hours later, she passed.

The Wish and Forgiveness Video

I have heard—and have had—many different types of conversations related to death and dying, in many ways, with many different kinds of people. We all have wishes and regrets—but not everyone is able to express them face-to-face. I have suggested to my own family and patients the idea of creating a "wish and forgiveness" video. These short, five-minute videos can produce a wealth of healing to the family members left behind so that prayer and unity can follow.

The wish and forgiveness video idea began with one of my patients. Hector was a sixty-five-year-old gentleman in the final stages of severe lung fibrosis—scar tissue in the lungs. The scar tissue was the result of a disease of unknown cause frequently called idiopathic pulmonary fibrosis (IPF). IPF had covered Hector's lungs with scar tissue. He required five liters of oxygen—an unusually massive amount—to maintain oxygen levels around 88 percent. I met Hector during his last hospitalization before passing. I walked into his room, and he was sitting up and breathing more than thirty-five times per minute (for comparison, normal respiratory rate is twelve to eighteen breaths per minute). His hair was wet, sweat was dripping from his forehead, and his hands were gripping and squeezing his knees. He was on the BiPAP twenty-four hours a day. He hadn't been able to talk for over a week. He had also decided against intubation.

Three years earlier, just after getting his IPF diagnosis, Hector joined the Pulmonary Fibrosis Foundation support group. He learned through this group that when he got to the point of persistent respiratory failure, intubation would not help him recover. His only option at that point would be a lung transplant, and he did not qualify for one due to his many medical problems.

I introduced myself and went through my list of questions about the disease and follow-up care. We talked about the fact that he was not eligible for a transplant. Hector mostly listened, until I asked about intubation. At that point, he quickly jumped and said, "You need to watch this video." It was Hector explaining what he wanted in terms of end-of-life care. He had recorded the video a year ago and had just recently updated it. I was impressed. I had never seen anyone go to those lengths before. I usually use my driving time to think, and on my way home that day, I was pondering how Hector's video had impacted me. I thought of one element that might make Hector's video even more profound—adding expressions of forgiveness, which are sometimes too hard to do face-to-face.

And so the wish and forgiveness video was born. I often suggest to patients that they make one. It's easy and can be done from a hospital bed. It doesn't need to be a professional production. Even a cell phone can serve as a recorder. The main idea is to express your last wishes to and for your family and friends and to share fears, regrets, and in some cases, apologies.

Family and friends who are left behind treasure wish and forgiveness videos. They are a meaningful tool for healing and something families can turn to during the grieving process, which has only just begun.

ACTION   Encourage a Conversation

Jot down a few statements you could use to start a conversation about life with your loved one. Example: "Mom, I'm so grateful for you. I hope you know I'm here for you."

Caring for You

Eat healthy foods. When you're running on adrenaline, it can be easy to forgo a healthy diet, and before long, you're feeling fatigued and ill. Instead of relying on vending machine snacks and hospital cafeterias, have food delivered to the hospital. Or ask a friend or your church family if they'd be willing to cook a few meals for you.

Main Chapter Takeaways

- Most people on their deathbed want to say something important before they die, and it's important that we be there to listen.

- Last conversations have a healing effect on patients and family—mentally, emotionally, physically, and spiritually.

- These profound conversations are often missed during the flurry of medical treatments and decisions. We must look for opportunities to have them.

- Reassuring and comforting patients makes it easier for them to begin these conversations under the stress of illness.

- Regrets, wishes for loved ones, and wisdom are the main topics.

- Patients, with the help of family, can make a wish and forgiveness video to better express themselves.

Grieving, Letting Go, and Acceptance

Lessons from the Orinoco

Along the northern shore of Venezuela toward the Atlantic Ocean, the delta of the Orinoco River branches off, producing sixty narrow waterways (*caños*) and forty rivers that diffuse through thirteen thousand miles of thickly forested islands, lagoons, canals, and swamps. The always-green, towering palm trees cover a fascinating reservoir of orchids, wild pineapples, grapes, plantains, and bromeliads (plants that take in their nutrients through their leaves instead of roots). The waterways are usually congested by a web of water hyacinth with a beautiful purple flower. The woodsy smell of moist earth combined with dry fallen leaves is the aromatherapy of the people who live here. This earthly fragrance penetrates the deepest part of the soul, producing a calming effect that only the Orinoco jungle can offer.

The Orinoco is the harmonious home of the Warao Indians and other groups, as well as a multitude of wildlife such as jaguars, pumas, red howler monkeys, manatees, and pink dolphins, just to mention a few. The rainbow of colors from parrots, toucans, falcons, harpy eagles, weaverbirds, and hummingbirds decorate the beauty of the forest.

Perhaps this heavenly habitat is the reason the Warao Indians have made this region their home for more than two thousand years. This community of about twenty thousand people has managed to preserve its ancient culture in spite of the encroachment of civilization in the form of oil wells, the hearts of palm business, and tourism. They have managed this in part because the delta they live in is so hard to reach. Although the waterways are navigable, dense tropical rain forests render it inaccessible by land.

In the Warao language, *Orinoco* means "a place to paddle," and *Warao* means "the boat people." Water is everywhere and a meaningful part of the Warao culture. They likely swim more than they walk (the shape of their feet attests to this, as they have maintained some distinctive weblike features), and they feel just as much at home in a canoe as in their shelters. The Orinoco Delta is also an area plagued by tuberculosis (TB).

An alarming number of Warao suffer from TB. Entire families, in fact. This serious bacterial infection usually invades the lungs, but it can attack other body parts as well. A fairly well-known case is author Thomas Wolfe, who died in 1938 from TB of the brain. In the United States, TB was prevalent until about 1947, when the antibiotic streptomycin was first introduced. If someone displayed symptoms of TB, they were quarantined or required to convalesce in a sanatorium for up to a year in order to heal. Time, medicine, and containment nearly eradicated the disease in the Western world. The Warao, however, do not have a clinic or a doctor trained in Western medicine to regularly test for and treat TB. And they do not have a facility in which to convalesce. Many of them are leery about going to the nearest city, where they could visit a clinic and receive the TB test and vaccine. And so 80 percent of the population is infected with TB, and 60 percent show symptoms. Approximately fifteen hundred children under five years of age die every year of multiple infectious diseases.[1] Dysentery and fever also take the lives of many Warao in Venezuela, where the infant mortality rate is an alarming 39 percent.[2]

Along with TB, these health concerns are so prevalent that Warao families do not name a child until he or she is at least six or seven years old, when the likelihood of survival is greater.

The prevalence of these health conditions stems in part from the Warao lifestyle. They live in wall-less, thatched-roof shelters built on large platforms made of tree trunks along the swampy shores. They pour their feces and urine into the river flowing underneath—the perfect habitat for parasites and bacteria and the same water they use to cook, drink, and bathe in.

At the age of twenty-six, while I was still living in Cuba, I was invited to conduct medical research in the Orinoco Delta, and of course I accepted. You can't imagine how excited I was as a young and energetic pulmonary resident. In addition to leaving my country for the first time in my life, I was going to make a difference in the lives of people who had little to no access to medical care. I was raring to go.

My charge was to go house to house and interview Warao families. I would also administer the purified protein derivative (PPD) skin test and return forty-eight hours later to determine whether anyone tested positive. Those with typical symptoms and a positive smear were to be treated, and all children would be vaccinated. A very organized person, I knew just what I would have to do to ensure my results would be valid. I couldn't wait to get started.

On the surface, this sounds like a simple job, right? Talk to nice people, inject 1 cc of PPD, and return to see how they are doing. But initially, this research project was one of the most frustrating of my life. As a scientist, I needed to record results. To do so, I needed names and to fill out paperwork. The beautiful and loving Warao did not live by my rules or paperwork or needs. A rich culture and strong community dictated their behaviors, not my pens and needles. The younger children didn't have names, and the moms didn't want to talk about illness in their family. Perhaps it was a self-protective measure.

My frustration ended the day I learned to treat my patients the way the anthropologists on my team treated them—the day I learned to embrace my patients for who they are. The anthropologists didn't come to the Warao to change them. They came to learn about them. These researchers didn't criticize or fight the Warao ways; they were enriched by their experience in the Orinoco. Once I was able to follow their lead, I changed my perspective from that of a conquistador to a compassionate caregiver, and my patients became my teachers. And in three short months, the Warao taught me more about death and grieving than I would have learned in a lifetime of trials.

A Modern Fear

Even with all the advances of medicine, no matter how far we advance scientifically, life is terminal. There is a limit to this life, and understanding that helps us frame the reality of facing our death and the deaths of those we love. In Western cultures, we struggle with the acceptance part. It's an ingrained fear, a fear that grows because we don't allow ourselves to talk about it. In truth, until we can accept that death is inevitable—that all of us must someday leave this earth plane—we do not let go. And letting go is the key to healing from the shock and dismay of losing a loved one.

The process of grieving is different for everyone—and every culture. In my practice, I see all types of reactions. Some people are truly angry and others depressed. All negative feelings—whether anger or anxiety or hatred—stem from fear. It's the same picture. Other limitations that I see are more culturally bound. Now that we live in a more global community, we must learn to be sensitive to how other cultures respond to grief.

The Warao grieve for a deceased loved one, but their perspective of death takes a 180-degree turn when compared to Western culture, and this seems to accelerate the grieving process.

It begins with a ceremony, much like any funeral. In accordance with tradition, the Warao use dugout canoes as coffins. Bodies are wrapped in hammocks, placed in the canoes, sealed in mud, and set upon stilts in a cemetery located just outside the village. For several days after someone dies, the Warao mourn for their loved one. They wail, and the men participate in some ceremonial drinking. They cry and feel sorrow. But the grieving process ends after two days maximum. It's not that they take death lightly. I tend to think their ability to let go so quickly is steeped in how they perceive death: instead of feeling as if someone has been taken from them, either by God, the universe, circumstances, or some other source, the Warao see death as a form of giving back to the earth. If you think about it, giving back can be another way of saying "letting go."

The Warao are also a very tight community. When someone dies, community members gather and go through the grieving process together. No one is isolated or left to cry on their own. I witnessed this many times when I was among the Warao. Over the seventeen months I was stationed there, nearly one hundred people died, usually from disease. The death of a child was more dramatic. The women crowded and wailed around the body lying on the floor of the house. The men seemed to be detached, distant, collected—more as an expression of manhood. The women also cried and wailed during the funeral, but a few days later, life went on as usual as the women were busy with the other children. Families didn't dwell on the loss. By taking fear out of the equation—and by mourning and releasing emotions as a community—the Warao from all accounts seemed to be able to get through the majority of their grieving process quickly. From their vantage, death gives. It doesn't take away.

Having this perspective is, of course, easier said than done, especially when it comes to losing a son or daughter.

Letting Go at Its Best—and Hardest

One of my patients back in the United States was a twenty-three-year-old named Sean who had muscular dystrophy (MD), a genetic disease that causes the muscles to waste away. In his case, the condition left him paralyzed and with lungs that became more compromised as he got older, creating a host of breathing problems.

The life span of someone with MD usually reaches only to the twenties or thirties. Fully aware of this fact, Sean's parents made every effort to enjoy his company. They dedicated their lives to their boy. When he went away to college, they went with him. His father sat through all of his classes, so he could take notes for Sean. Both parents worked nights in order to support the family. They were an amazing family that many at our hospital found inspirational.

Now in his twenties, it was apparent Sean's time on earth was coming to an end. He began to visit the emergency room more frequently, with high levels of carbon dioxide in his blood, an indication that his muscles were weak and fatigued. During his last visit, he was taken to the ICU in a coma and with multi-organ failure, wholly dependent on machines to keep him among the living. With a heavy heart, I had to tell his wonderful, loving parents that their son had almost no chance of recovery.

We discussed the option of doing CPR if Sean stopped breathing. CPR, I explained to this distraught mother and father, wouldn't change the outcome of his case. We might break his ribs, and in his fragile state, this would probably cause a great deal of suffering, which we would be unable to address.

As we talked, they cried. I remember the gut-wrenching feeling of having nothing to offer them. This was a case where medicine in all its modern glory had no options left.

As the parents composed themselves, they talked about how they knew their son would have a short life from the moment he was born. They had decided from the beginning that they would fight for him as long as they could—but that when the time came, and they had done all they could, they would let Sean go with grace and dignity.

These amazing parents went into their dying son's room for the last time and talked to him for a long while. He was in a coma, and we can't be certain he was able to hear them, but the parents were not concerned with that. The act of talking to him seemed almost more important than whether he was able to take in what they were saying. I believe, in these cases, these conversations are highly therapeutic for the parents.

When they came out of Sean's room, they told us they wanted his suffering to end and for him to die in peace. He passed away in the ICU a few hours later.

There is pain in letting go. As a doctor and as a human being, I know this. The pain seems to come from everywhere and attack every part of our being: the gut-wrenching ache, the mental anguish, the emotional distress. What do we do with this pain? How do we get through it? How do we release it? What do we need to understand about it? We can't go back and change what happened. What can we do?

One thing I know for certain is that the experience of grieving is different for everyone. For some, it's a purely spiritual thing. For others, it is highly emotional or strictly rational. And for many, I suspect, it is a delicate dance of spirit, emotion, and reason. We may never fully understand why we must go through the grieving process or why it's sometimes so hard to let go. But grieve we must. One consequence of not grieving is depression, a low-grade funk we can't seem to pinpoint or feelings of despair, anxiety, and in many cases, physical illness.

The Consequences of Holding On

Alexander was laid up in a long-term care facility after having had a stroke from which he'd suffered a multitude of complications, including kidney failure requiring dialysis, respiratory failure that left him dependent on mechanical ventilation (a breathing machine), and heart failure. On top of that, his weakened immune system could not fight infection, and so he endured one infectious process after another. Alexander remained on a respirator until he died six months later in that facility. Vera, his beloved wife, had stayed at his bedside 24/7.

I was not in the hospital the week that Alexander passed, and I did not see Vera again until about five months later, when she came to my office as a patient. Vera came to me complaining of shortness of breath. She had been seen by many doctors, including cardiologists and pulmonologists, but no one could find anything physically wrong with her. She had every single test done, and all of the doctors concurred that her shortness of breath was related to anxiety and depression. She wanted another opinion.

I could rerun all the tests and repeat the exams the other doctors had done, but it was highly unlikely that my test results would vary from the many other test results I saw in her chart. Certainly, doctors miss diagnoses, but the chance that a dozen or so specialists would all miss a heart or lung condition was next to zero. Vera was a worrier by nature. This I knew from the time I'd spent with her while her husband was ill. Worry can transport us to the most uncomfortable mental state if we allow our thoughts to carry us there. So, like the anthropologists in the Orinoco, I took the approach of embracing

Vera for who she was and where she was in her grieving process. Unlike the other doctors Vera saw, I knew some of her history. And so Vera and I talked for at least a couple of hours. We talked mostly about what her life was like since Alexander had passed.

Vera was still living in the neighborhood she'd been in for twenty years, but she didn't get out much. Vera spoke broken English; her native language was Russian. Language barriers kept her from interacting with people she could relate to. Her daughter was a flight attendant and lived in another city. Her son lived nearby, but he was busy with work. He came to visit Vera once a week, usually for an hour or two on the weekend. She had no other family members and few friends. She didn't drive. Alexander had done the driving. These factors all contributed to her isolation, but more than that, Vera was still grieving deeply.

"How have you been feeling since Alexander passed?" I asked. She informed me that she still carried vivid images of his last days in the hospital, which were traumatic. Her mind kept going back to how he struggled—he would fight the breathing machine and choke on his mucus when phlegm entered the tube. When that happened, she was afraid he was going to suffocate and would call out for help. These memories were recycling through her mind, getting stronger instead of fading. Vera had become emotionally attached to the pain of her husband's experience, and she couldn't stop her thoughts. My belief is that Vera did not open herself up to the grieving process. She didn't fully accept her husband's death. She was in disbelief. The more she thought about it, the worse she felt.

If we don't allow ourselves to grieve, we create deep wounds that can add to our burden and hinder normal functionality. Vera repeatedly told me that life for her didn't have any more meaning because Alexander was gone. I talked to her about the community of ethnic Russians who lived close to her neighborhood. "Go there and try to make some friends. See if you can find someone who comes from your area in Russia, someone you can sit and talk to," I said. "Being with people who understand you and who will listen to you will help you release some of the mental burden. Conversations like these help you to let go."

I also tell family members and patients such as Vera that the key here is to keep your mind occupied, to find activities or hobbies that you can use to steer your thoughts away from the continuous recycling of images, over and over, in your brain. Removing yourself from your thoughts, getting absorbed in a project of some sort, is an excellent way to help get your mind in a healthier place. Anything that forces you to look outside of yourself helps—having a conversation means you sometimes have to listen, volunteering puts the focus on others, and getting involved in a project requires you to pay attention to what you're doing in the moment.

I believe wholeheartedly that medication may be needed for grieving people in some instances, particularly when someone is suffering from severe depression or anxiety, but I also believe that medication is not the real answer. The real answer is developing coping strategies. Those are developed by building relationships and interacting with other people.

After talking with Vera, I decided to do some tests and give her the second opinion she came in for, even though I was convinced that her symptoms were related to her husband's death. She was still vehemently attached to the grieving process. In some ways, it kept her husband near. I believed that her shortness of breath would resolve when she took care of herself emotionally, when she opened up to the grieving process.

I also recommended that she visit a psychologist, which she resisted until I said we could find one who spoke Russian, and then I directed her to my office assistant for help.

Research shows that the grieving process is expedited when people have the opportunity to talk, interact, and occupy their mind. For many people, the inability to move past their grief is due to the pain of letting go, a feeling that they are either responsible or guilty of something that they didn't do for their loved one. *I didn't do what I was supposed to do. Why didn't I do this? Why didn't I do that?* Most people go through this to some degree, but when people stay in that place, they spiral downward and can't help themselves. People need support to move beyond these thoughts.

Acceptance versus Denial

The Warao see a lot of death, but I don't believe this has made them immune to the emotional effects of it. Maybe it has made them efficient grievers, if there's such a thing. If anything, they have learned how to fully accept death. It's a part of their culture. They don't fight it, nor do they blame anyone for it. If I had to put my finger on it, I would say they forgo the experience of denial. Denial in our culture is fairly common. It's our way of protecting ourselves from what we don't want to feel or believe or have to give up. Denial and disbelief probably keep more people in the throes of grief than anything else. Yet, every now and then, denial opens the door to truth. It comes and goes, and when it pulls back like the tide, it gives us permission to feel again.

Denial is many times linked to blaming, and people can be quick to blame anyone in their path—the system, doctors, families, friends. When it comes to death, denial can be overpowering. We don't want to die, and we don't want to deal with dying. But we also don't want to be responsible for the death of anyone. I think that is probably an intrinsic human behavior. We don't want to be responsible, so it is easy to blame or pass on that responsibility to someone else, even when we know deep down that we're not speaking the truth. Negligence on the part of medical teams certainly exists, but for the great majority of people, most institutions go above and beyond to help their patients. Even then, people find space to blame.

Ms. Joanne Cummings's Case

Joanne Cummings was eighty-nine years old when she suffered a massive bleed to her brain, the result of high blood pressure. Large intracranial bleeds trigger massive inflammation and affect brain functioning. Her brain had lost its ability to communicate with the nerve centers in the lungs and airways. She was placed on a breathing machine. A brain scan showed bleeding plus a possible brain mass, or tumor. A chest scan revealed a mass in the right upper lung with evidence that it had spread to her spine. After two weeks in the ICU, a tracheostomy was performed. She then proceeded to develop one complication after another—a blood clot in the lower extremities, renal failure, ventilator-associated pneumonia, and a stomach bleed from the blood thinner she was taking.

Joanne had four children—a daughter and three sons. The daughter, Gracie, was always by her mother's bedside, taking care of all details. I met her when Joanne was transferred to the LTAC facility. Gracie slept in the hospital every night and paid a nurse assistant to be with her mom during the day until Gracie came back from work. Her siblings lived out of state, one in North Carolina and two in California. During a three-month period, I met only one of the sons face-to-face. That was the day he and his brothers fired all the doctors and called our team for a second opinion.

Gracie was embarrassed and ashamed of her brothers' behavior. They called regularly, complaining about nurses not responding to them, the food, the toothpaste, the English proficiency of the staff—you name it. Gracie, on the other hand, was so happy with the care provided that she praised the team regularly and constantly apologized for her brothers' behavior. She mentioned to us several times that her mom did not want to depend on life support, but she wanted to wait until her brothers had come to terms with the situation. Four months later, after watching her mother suffer from a multitude of complications, Gracie decided to call hospice and asked her brothers to come to see their mother before the transfer. They came, and Joanne passed away in hospice within hours of her transfer. All of her children were around her, but her sons were not really with her. They were still blaming everyone for their mother's death.

Gracie understood how advanced and terminal her mother's condition was. The last time I saw her, she told me, "Dr. Ferrer, I have enjoyed living with my mom, going on cruises together, and opening a business, and caring for her. She was always there for me, and I wanted to be here for her. Thank you for all you did to make her comfortable."

Letting Go Is a Spiritual Act

When I was a pulmonary and critical care fellow at George Washington University, my cotrainees—the residents and fellows under my tutelage in the ICU—had one goal: they didn't want anyone to die on their shift. Shifts for these young residents lasted twelve hours. Yet, without fail, this was their fear. By the end of their three-year residency, some had learned to deal with death, but others remained distant and detached. That's a long time to harbor such a fear when you're training to be a doctor.

When I'm in the ICU, which I consider my "stage," where I'm acting and teaching at the same time, every time I hear that fear, I try to explore it deeply with my residents and fellows. They know that I like to go deep. "Why do you react that way?" I ask. I hear a plethora of answers, usually wrapped up in the beliefs from their upbringing.

Even when we know that a patient is going to die, we fight and fight against this unseen enemy because we don't want to face the experience. That phenomenon has influenced the way I see letting go. Today, I think more about the patient and the family than about the system and what I think is right or wrong, and this brings me back to embracing them.

In some ways, I believe a doctor is a soldier, a soldier fighting this unseen enemy of death. I have to guide my patients away from doubts and misconceptions. I have the tremendous privilege to guide and protect patients and families from the deep emotional scars that can come from the fear of dying. I have to be impartial and nonjudgmental at the same time. I have to exercise the habit of being present and being there for the family, to focus on what they need and know that there is a healing that will have to take place when the patient dies. There is a healing process that we, as providers, have the privilege to be a part of. When families are able to let go, the medical team feels it as well. It's a constellation of ripple effects.

I have seen various cultures face death totally differently, but I see that families who have a deep understanding of life or religion tend to be more graceful and understanding. They don't tend to fight against the deep emotional winds that can be stirred up during this process. For the great majority of people, being with death is more spiritual than anything else. Deeply pragmatic people or the people who are totally materialistic miss the spiritual opportunity before them, but in all my years of practicing, I've only met a handful of people like that. Most people realize that at the end of life, they are in the presence of something deeply important and with great meaning.

The great meaning of life is in what we don't see. I have experienced a variety of reactions from people in trying to explain that spiritual connection. Some people cry, others smile, for some a cold emptiness fills the room, and some have a deep sense of peace that you can feel.

As for Me . . .

The other day, I was driving my kids to school when my youngest daughter said, "Daddy, we have a kid in my classroom that is just like you!"

"How so?" I asked, not really sure if I wanted to hear the answer.

"He can make a life lesson out of anything!"

And so I guess it's apparent to my family at least that part of my healing involves finding the silver lining. Anyone who works in an ICU is pretty tough. They witness death on a daily basis and absorb the grief and sometimes the hysteria. It's impossible not to. So medical staff needs to heal too. We must let go daily. If we didn't, we'd likely burn out within a couple of years on the job.

As for me, I find a daily reprieve. I like to pray and run and find interesting things to do, and I have found a little bit of refuge in writing—that's the reason I began to collect the stories you are reading in this book, and hundreds more.

ACTION   Try Guided Imagery

Guided imagery, or visualization, can be a pleasant way to practice letting go. You can find many guided imagery CDs or YouTube videos online.

Caring for You

Grieving can be physically exhausting. Burke, a friend of the family, developed chronic fatigue for six months after losing her father. She told me once that she felt as tired as if she had had the flu for months.

What activities take you to your happy place? Think about activities that you become totally absorbed in, so much that they take your mind off of everything else: running, golfing, sewing, gardening, playing music, playing cards, writing, meditating, praying. Write them down and make a point to do one of them every day.

Main Chapter Takeaways

- There is no right or wrong way to grieve. What's most important is that we allow ourselves to grieve.

- Effects of not grieving can include depression, anxiety, and physical illness.

- Talking through our grief with supportive people, helping other people, and occupying ourselves with hobbies are helpful. Prayer, meditation, and exercise are also valuable.

Post-Death Paperwork

Funerals, Taxes, Passwords, and More

Far too soon after a loved one passes, families are asked to park their grief as they're launched into the practicalities of life. For many people, it is difficult, impossible even, to shift gears and move from the depth of emotion to what now seem like distant and trivial details, such as paying a mortgage or answering an email. Granted, there are also people who find these responsibilities to be just the distraction they need at the moment. They excel during a crisis, as resiliency swiftly moves them into action. Whatever category you fall into, you need to know where to start. What do you do after a loved one dies?

Family members of my patients frequently tell me they are at a loss. They don't know what to do, what to tell loved ones, where to make funeral arrangements. Resources to help manage what comes next are few and far between, so I've included this chapter to help guide you through the process. This chapter offers a series of lists and scripts I've refined over the years to help families through the process of tying up loose ends, which are usually more numerous than we imagine. And some, if overlooked, can create complications down the road, such as ignoring an open bank account with monthly fees or failing to pay back taxes on a home.

Every family has at least a few tasks to consider:

- Arranging the funeral

- Informing family and friends

- Contacting Social Security and Medicare

- Changing advance directives (of a surviving spouse, for example)

- Closing bank accounts

- Selling the car and other assets that require a death certificate, title, or authentication

- Paying bills and canceling credit cards and other accounts

- Accessing online accounts

- Dealing with email and social media accounts

- Canceling monthly subscriptions and services

- Dealing with taxes—the one thing that almost certainly outlives us all

Calling each of these "tasks" is an understatement, as each usually involves multiple steps—searching for paperwork and contact information, making phone calls, preparing to-do lists, filling out paperwork. Many of these jobs involve coordinating doctors, lawyers, accountants, and other specialists. Most of them require making decisions—some of them minor, others that feel monumental. Some of them even require resolving conflict. As a doctor, I wasn't particularly concerned with any of these matters—that is, until I met Margarita.

Ms. Margarita Hernandez's Case

Five years ago marked an important change in my life, and it all started with Margarita Hernandez. Margarita's husband, Marcus, was very sick, in and out of the ICU. Every time he went to a regular floor in the hospital, he would come back to the ICU within the next day or two with his lungs full of fluid. This condition, called pulmonary edema, results when a heart is too weak to pump all the blood received with each contraction, and the lungs end up filling with all the blood that the heart is unable to pump. Pulmonary edema is easy to recognize in heart patients. When fluid fills the lungs, they sit up suddenly gasping for air and reaching for the oxygen with trembling hands. Margarita had seen this happen to her husband multiple times. Each time, she felt traumatized and unable to shake the image from her head.

In the ICU, our medical team once again put him through the motions—electrodes on his chest, oxygen mask, nurses drawing blood, respiratory therapist piercing a needle into his wrist in search of arterial blood to measure blood oxygen levels, BiPAP machine, nurses giving furosemide (the IV form of the water pill), all while Marcus struggled with every breath. I was then called in to Marcus's room.

I walked quickly past Margarita, who was standing outside the ICU room, trembling but hopeful, waiting for the team to finish stabilizing Marcus. She later told me she held her breath while the team was in the room. In the past, it had always worked; inevitably, the doctor would come out of the ICU and tell her, "*Está mejor* [He is better]. We put him on the breathing machine."

I opened Marcus's mouth and slid the laryngoscope between his tongue and palate and then pulled the base of his tongue up and forward with my left hand until I saw the voice box. Using my right hand, and carefully protecting his upper teeth and lips, I passed the endotracheal tube through the vocal cords into the windpipe, or trachea. I have done this procedure thousands of times, yet I still hold my breath, zero in, mentally cancel out all noises, and pray that it doesn't end up in the food pipe instead of the windpipe. When I saw the tube passing through Marcus's vocal cords, I knew it was in the windpipe, and I could breathe again.

"Inflate the tube balloon and bag him," I told the respiratory therapist. I carefully watched for his chest to rise as she squeezed the bag. I put my stethoscope on the left side of his chest and waited for the gush of air as the therapist squeezed the bag, then repeated the same ritual on the right side. Within minutes, Marcus was connected to the ventilator, a compressor that pumped air into Marcus's lungs at a set volume and rate.

The monitor showed normal heart waves at a rate of sixty beats per minute, but his blood pressure was barely detectable. My fingers reached for the right side of his neck, then the left, then his groin.

"No pulse, no pulse! Call Code Blue," I shouted. In no time, Cathy, Marcus's nurse, punched the Code Blue button located on the wall directly behind his bed.

Code Blue is a standard hospital emergency code. When Cathy pushed the button, she activated the overhead call system that blares "Code Blue" throughout the hospital. This announcement mobilizes a team of nurses, doctors, and respiratory therapists to the room where the call was initiated.

Margarita did not speak English, but she fully understood the call for Code Blue. She had remained by Marcus's bedside on every trip he had to the ICU, making only short trips to the hospital cafeteria for coffee or something to eat. She would jump every time she heard "Code Blue" if she wasn't by his side.

Now, outside the ICU, she waited patiently for the bed number. This time she heard "Code Blue ICU4." Standing outside the room, she looked up and saw the number "4" by the side of Marcus's door—then a flurry of activity. Nurses pushed in the "crash cart" that holds a defibrillator on top. Nurses, respiratory therapist, residents, and students ran past Margarita—all focused intently on Marcus's cardiac arrest. Nobody stopped to talk to Margarita, much less comfort her.

Forty-five minutes later, I came out of the room, sweating, pulling off my gloves in slow motion, searching for a family member. Behind me came the students and residents with sober faces, faces of defeat. I put my right hand on Margarita's shoulder and told her, "*Lo siento* [I'm sorry]. He passed. We did all we could."

"*Yo sé, Doctor* [I know, Doctor]," she said.

Shortly afterward, I pronounced his death on paper, citing the code "99239," a number I know all too well. He was dead, and there was nothing more I could do except to cite the appropriate insurance billing code and initiate the issuing of the death certificate, a document I knew Margarita would need to get her affairs in order. All the paperwork was complete when I, very simply and directly, asked Margarita if she knew what she was going to do next. Her eyes welled up with water. She was clearly distraught over her husband's death, but underneath her tears lay her most profound communication: Margarita was not only heartbroken, she was utterly and unabashedly confused.

I let her cry for about a minute, and then asked her again, "Do you know what you are going to do next?"

"*No lo sé* [I don't know]," she said. Adding to her confusion was the fact that she only spoke Spanish. My heart reached out to her. I felt equally lost just seventeen years prior, when I landed in the United States for the first time. I was a Cuban defector, placed on a plane by a group of friends in Venezuela, and headed for Atlanta. I had $80 in my pocket and didn't speak a word of English. I was also traumatized by my experiences during the escape. If it weren't for the kind woman standing behind me at the airline ticket counter, I wouldn't have had the extra $100 I needed to buy a ticket for Miami, where my host family, old neighbors of my family in Cuba, was waiting for me. (That family, by the way, had a daughter named Nikki, who would become my beloved wife.)

Kind gestures go a long way. This I fully understood. So when Margarita told me she had no idea what she or the hospital was going to be doing next, I paused long enough to recognize that, despite my busy schedule, she needed my help. The problem was that I also had no clue what happened next. So I went and talked to the chart nurses, and I went and talked to people who were on call in the ICU. Surprise, surprise—everyone was in the same boat, passing the buck on to the funeral homes or to the medical examiner. I realized that no one in the hospital fully understood what happens after our jobs of trying to save lives were done. If my staff and I were confused, imagine how a grief-stricken woman who didn't speak English and had no family or friends to help her felt. She was in confused waters, being tossed in every direction, with no idea how to move forward.

After half an hour, I had no answers, but I couldn't just walk away or refer her to someone who would most likely turn around and refer her to someone else. So I did a little research.

I spent the next few hours of my time in the ICU reaching out to people. I called several funeral homes and the medical examiner and did some searching on the Internet. The people I spoke with gave me very structured answers, as if they were reading directly from an instruction manual, similar to how a flight attendant might announce safety precautions at the beginning of a flight. Each person read their script, but I was left hanging with more questions than answers.

"I'm trying to help a lady with no family, who doesn't speak English," I quickly added. Then the answers were more explicit. I put together a short list of things that needed to be done:

1. Call Martinez Funeral Home and ask for Carlos.

2. Determine if cremation is an option.

3. Ask if she wants a funeral service.

4. . . .

Extracting the right information from my sources seemed to take forever. The ICU, for some mysterious reason, was unusually quiet. I thank God that I had time to help Margarita, for guilt would not allow me to let her figure it out by herself. She reminded me almost too much of my mom, who also does not speak English despite attempting to learn it at the age of seventy-nine, bless her heart. But my mom, like Margarita, also has no idea how the system works, so much so that even checking in at a doctor's appointment is a major ordeal.

Margarita looked at me with a half-smile every time I lifted my head from the phone across the other side of the nursing station counter. She was in deep pain but pulled what she could from her emotional bank to communicate her appreciation. I imagine I offered the same tender expression to the lady who helped me in the Atlanta airport years earlier. I did not register that moment in my memory bank, at least not consciously.

I handed my short list of tasks, written neatly in Spanish, to Margarita. "Do you have a family or a friend who can help you through this?"

"*Pues no . . . usted, Doctor* [No, just you, Doctor]."

"Thank you. I love that. But you need somebody to help you navigate through this system."

"*Sí, en la iglesia* [Yes, at church]."

I called Miriam, Margarita's church friend, and explained the situation. Miriam also only spoke Spanish, but luckily she had two bilingual daughters who could help.

I felt Margarita's love when she hugged me tight in her arms.

Becoming Part of the Solution

In the preface, I talk about how I made a conscious decision to stop viewing death as a failure and start tending to the living. Death is not a failure. Refusing to get involved in the process is. When I say, "Do you know what you want to do? I want to help you. Is there anyone you'd like me to call?" I open the door not only to an important conversation but to healing. When families feel this support, they feel the compassion. In my experience, compassion alters, if even only slightly, every sad situation for the better. And it always points in the direction of healing.

Study after study supports the fact that when someone dies in an institution, most nurses, doctors, and people around the patient do not know what they should do.[1] Only 1 to 2 percent of the families I talk to clearly know what to do. I, for one, did not know until I met Margarita. People who know what to do usually have a plan that the deceased person left behind, with a clear description of what he or she wants for a funeral and the estate or belongings—a solid plan. But very few people really have everything thought out. Most people believe that if they have purchased a plot in a cemetery, that's all they need. But that's simply not true anymore.

So I usually wait for a few minutes, and then I ask the family that key question: "Do you know what you are going to do next? Do you understand what the next step is?" On occasion, I get an "Oh, yes!" But very seldom do I hear those words. If the answer is something like, "Yes, he wants to be cremated and for us to keep his ashes on the mantel. We will have a ceremony in July, when everyone in the family can be present," then I leave the family to take care of matters.

If I see that all is not well organized, I take the liberty of offering some advice. "You know, it's important that you reach out to people who will help you. You need support. You're going to be responsible for a lot of things over the next few weeks, and it's important to reach out to someone who can help you. Do you want me to call someone in your family or a friend?" Most people, I would estimate nine out of ten, respond "yes." They usually give me a number for someone they know who will help them. In many cases, people want me to call a family member they haven't spoken to in years—usually an estranged sibling.

These calls take time, but they bring empathy and healing to the conversation quickly. When feeling loss, the fragility of life is palpable. People feel the time they've wasted fighting. The death of a loved one can sometimes serve to bring families closer—even long-time rivals like Michael and Johnny.

The Smart Thing to Do

One of my patients was a professor who died of lung cancer produced by his longstanding smoking habit. He had two very intelligent sons. Michael was a professor at a local college and the other son, Johnny, was an engineer. The two siblings had been fighting since their mother died, about six or seven years prior to their father's death. Michael had been very involved in caring for his father. In fact, he was the only person involved. Our medical team, including myself, had no idea Johnny even existed. When his father died, Michael passed me a handwritten note with Johnny's number. He said Johnny was his brother, and he asked me to call him.

I dialed Johnny's number, introduced myself, and explained that his father was in the hospital and that he had just passed. Johnny immediately started screaming on the phone, and I explained that I was really sorry, but I didn't know that my patient had another son. So he went on ranting about his brother. He said a lot of negative things about Michael, who was standing right next to me within earshot, and Michael heard the screaming and yelling as I pulled the phone off my ear. The expletives were flying left and right, and then all of a sudden, Johnny stopped, and that's when his brother asked me for the phone.

"Johnny, it's your brother. It's over. We need to talk. We need to put a stop to this. We, too, are going to die." The two nurses next to us started crying as these two guys began reconnecting. They talked about miscommunication and how they were feeling. In this phone conversation, they began tearing down the wall they had built between them. It was as if the death of their father shone a light on their behavior. It was very touching for all of us to hear. "It's over. We need to fix it."

Emotion is a part of all the calls I make on behalf of someone who just lost a loved one and must contact someone they haven't talked to in years. Johnny expressed anger initially. Most of the time, people either cry, scream, or curse. I always give them a little bit of time. There is a tremendous power in a pause and silence, and so I use it. When they ask me, "Are you there? What should we do next?" I try to communicate that life is fragile and that it's important to reach out to your family because they want to talk to you. Most of the time, at the end of the conversation, people recognize the need to do something, to move one step closer to reconciliation or something else.

The next step is just as big. It requires considering your loved one's last wishes.

Last Wishes

When making funeral arrangements, the best place to start is to consider what is known about the deceased's wishes—or what you imagine they'd be. This can open up a detailed conversation among family members, and the wishes people come up with determine all of the steps that follow. I usually find that the more people involved, the better, as everyone seems to be able to contribute memories that help to piece together a puzzle. These conversations also have a way of grounding everyone.

General David White's Case

Retired army general David White was eighty years old when I met him in the ICU after he'd had a stroke. A diabetic, he had suffered major damage to most of his organs, resulting in chronic heart failure, renal failure, amputation below the left knee, and multiple small strokes. Still, he remained clear minded.

When I entered his room, I found General David sitting up in bed hooked to a monitor through a web of cables. I rolled the curtain aside, and he put down his newspaper. He looked straight at me through his thick glasses, gasped for air, and with shortness of breath, told me: "Here I . . . am . . . again, Dr. Ferrer . . . with another stroke . . . but I'm still standing . . . until . . . my last breath."

I caught myself taking deep breaths, as if I wanted to breathe for him. I was also tempted to instruct him not to talk, but I held my peace. He needed to be heard. Within minutes, his son and daughter walked into the room, followed by the general's girlfriend.

"Dr. Ferrer . . . I'm glad . . . you are here," he said, sitting upright with his neck stretched out and shoulders held back in a perfect military posture. "I want to . . . explain to you and . . . my family . . . my wishes." His shaky hands waved a few pieces of paper he had next to him.

"Why do you do that, Dad?" said his daughter, looking at the "get well" balloon next to window. "You are a fighter. You will, once again, get out of here."

"Yes, Dad. What do you want to do when we get home? I thought about going fishing," his son added. As he spoke, his eyes moved toward the window. The conversation seemed to take him out of his comfort zone. The general's girlfriend didn't say anything. She stood in the corner in silence. She seemed to be waiting to see how the conversation would unfold.

"Listen . . . *Listen to me!* . . . ," a longer pause. "My precious family . . . I love you all . . . and because . . . I love you . . . we need to talk about the end. . . . I know what will happen . . . if we don't have this . . . unpleasant talk."

General David went on to explain how he came to terms with death years ago while fighting in Vietnam. He saw many friends die, each of them a reminder of his own mortality. He learned firsthand that you have to let your loved ones know your wishes.

He went on to explain to the family what they would inherit. He also outlined his wishes for a funeral, the hymn to be sung at the church, where to find his military uniform, people to call, the bank representative's number, his accountant's contact number, his email addresses, charitable contributions he wanted to make, and information for the bank account he opened with $10,000 for his funeral. He had already calculated the cost of finger food for after the church service, adding $2,000 to account for inflation. General David then pronounced that he was DNR and asked to be placed in hospice.

Although awkward in the beginning, the conversation turned into a wonderful experience. Instead of trying to convince their father that he shouldn't talk about his death, the kids accepted his wishes. They listened, and he felt heard. The next day, when I walked into his room, he told me, "I have found . . . peace . . . peace . . . all around. . . . Thank you." I felt it as well. A tremendous sense of peace filled his room. Days later, he passed comfortably in the hospital.

I've heard many of these conversations over the years, and they tend to be somber, as the focus is solely on the deceased's last wishes. Not a single ego is willing to penetrate and alter this mood, which seems to come from a place of surrender. It's reinforced by the group, the family's collective grief. And there's a peace about it that's hard to describe. The closest I come is to say it feels like all resistance has completely dissolved, leaving only acceptance.

Exploring Last Wishes

A few simple questions can start the conversation about last wishes, if these weren't determined before your loved one passed. People will start recalling information about one topic or another, and soon the next steps become clear. You will likely come up with many more questions, but these will give you a good start:

- Did she want to be cremated?
- Did she have a favorite dress she'd like to be buried in?

- Would she want any special items with her?
- Did she request certain makeup?
- What was her favorite flower?
- Did she leave an address book with people to contact?
- Did he say he wanted a simple ceremony?
- Did he say he wanted a big celebration?
- What was his favorite place in the world?
- Would he want us to spread his ashes there?
- Should we plan to gather at his favorite restaurant? ✑

A Sample To-Do List

Once families have sorted through last wishes, the work of pulling it all together begins. This is not something you'll want to do by yourself, if at all possible. There is a power behind asking for help, and there's no shame in doing so. And so reaching out to someone on the medical team is the number one item on the to-do list I've created for you.

The following tasks are best taken care of by the family Leader, the health-care agent, attorney-in-fact, or the person closest to the deceased. *Always* ask for help.

- Ask the medical team for guidance.

- Ask a support person (family member/friend) for help.

- Notify immediate family members.

- Arrange the funeral.

- Inform other family and friends.

- Notify your employer and your loved one's employer.

- Acquire the death certificate.

- Look for important paperwork.

Ask the Medical Team for Guidance

If you've established a relationship with the medical team, asking them for help will be easy. If you haven't had a chance to know the team, or relationship building has not been easy, asking for help might feel awkward, but if you're confused, don't hesitate to ask *someone.*

Ask a Support Person (Family Member/Friend) for Help

I see many family members who are so grief-stricken that they find it hard to talk. If you need moral support, that is your first task. If you can't think clearly enough, ask a nurse to help you make the phone call. If you're the type of person who doesn't need moral support, at least plan on doing some delegating. Funeral arrangements, for instance, involve several steps, from picking out the funeral parlor to selecting a grave marker. The family may have already decided how much to spend on a coffin or what kind of flowers to buy, but someone still has to do the legwork. In my years of practice, I have found that most people are willing to help. Even the busiest of families understand that when someone dies, it's time to be present and help.

Notify Immediate Family Members

Today we have so many ways to get in touch and connect with one another. Most people have electronic relationships (Facebook, Instagram), and those are good, but when a loved one passes, there is no substitute for an in-person conversation with family. Many people find it difficult to reach out to family because oftentimes they haven't talked to an immediate family member in years. This is just another reality modern life has brought to us all. So don't be afraid to call your family. We all share the same guilt of not having been in touch. Texting is a cold approach for emotional news such as a death. An in-person visit or a phone call is the best way to communicate the news. If you cannot make the phone call, ask someone on the medical team or your support person to do it for you.

⚘ To Post or Not to Post?

These days, it's common to hear about a death over Facebook.
Common courtesy dictates that an old high school friend should not
find out about the death before your siblings do. All immediate family
members should be told the news as soon as possible and before
people learn about it through social media. Make sure everyone
understands this, especially teenagers who might be quick to post
and not understand the emotional repercussions for family members.
Once all immediate family members, employers, and as many
extended family, close friends, and neighbors as possible have been
notified, it's appropriate to share the news on social media. ⤸

Arrange for the Funeral

I usually tell people that, when you contact funeral homes, be careful
with the checklist they are going to send you. After reading it, you
might feel so overwhelmed that you won't sleep at night. I always
suggest dividing up the list and tackling it in phases. The first phase
should be dealing with what you are going to do now. The second
phase is what you are going to do a week from today. Also, be careful
when choosing products and options. Costs can add up quickly, and
emotions and guilt can drive you to spend more than you'd planned
on. Family members should agree in advance on how much to spend.
For most families, this amount is dependent on a life insurance
policy or an amount set aside by the deceased for this purpose. Try to
approach the purchase as you would any other major expense. Stick
to the budget and remember that you must be accountable to the rest
of the family. And read the fine print. Discuss, make a plan, pause,
take a deep breath—and read the fine print.

⚘ Basic Checklist for a Funeral

Some funeral homes provide a twenty-five-item checklist. Here's a
simplified version. Funeral parlor directors can help you get through
all of these steps.

Letter or Email Communicating the Death. Most people today are moving away from newspaper obituaries for two reasons: One, it can be expensive ($280–$600) and, two, most people don't read them.

Cemetery Plot Location. If you know that a cemetery plot has been purchased but can't find the paperwork, call the cemetery directly.

Type of Memorial Service. How you handle the memorial service is very personal. What would the deceased want? You can have a religious, military, nondenominational, or fraternal service. Decide whether you want to include photos, videos, music, and so on. You only have so much time to prepare. It is more than acceptable to keep it simple. Again, ask for help.

Flowers versus Donations. Most families go by their loved one's wishes. If he or she was devoted to a certain charity, you might request that people donate to the charity in lieu of sending flowers.

Eulogies. Select the speakers to best represent your loved one. If you are going to hold a eulogy, ask the speaker(s) as soon as possible, so they have time to prepare a speech that truly honors your loved one. In my hometown of Guantánamo, there was a guy known for just adding the name of the deceased person to the same speech he gave each time. People knew what he was going to say before he said it.

Guest Book and Funeral Program. Options these days include a printed program and guest book. You can also opt to collect and store electronic condolences in a folder (label it "Guest Book"), including those that come via a social media site, the funeral home's online condolences, or to your personal email.

Cremation? What Will You Do with the Ashes? Cremation has become more and more popular. Some people bury the ashes in a cemetery plot. Others spread all or a portion of them somewhere special or keep them in an urn.

Date of the Service. Funerals usually take place a few days after the death. These days, visitation is usually short—sometimes only a few hours—or limited to close family. It's not uncommon for people in their eighties or nineties to have already lost most of their peers. Even big families lean toward shorter visitation periods. With cremation, services can be held at any time. Some families wait for a special date (birthday, anniversary) or when they know all of the family can gather for a ceremony. ⬿

Cremation: More Popular Than Ever

The number of people in the United States choosing cremation over a traditional burial has been steadily increasing in recent years, from 26.2 percent in 2000 to 48.6 percent in 2015. By 2020, more than half of Americans are expected to be cremated.

You likely won't want to arrange cremation for a loved one who hasn't requested it. Although cremation is as old as time, it defies tradition in the United States. For some people, that's the appeal—a more personalized approach to a burial.

Following are some of the top reported reasons people are choosing cremation:

Cost. Cremation is about half the price of average burial and funeral costs (although prices for urns range between $100 and $2,000).

Simplicity. There are no pallbearers or caskets; gravesites and headstones are optional.

Flexibility. The ceremony can be postponed to accommodate schedules.

Personalization. The ceremony can be individualized (ashes spread over a mountaintop or in a sea).

Proximity. Ashes can remain close to family members in an urn. ⬿

Inform Other Family and Friends

Anyone who was close to the deceased either now or in the recent past should be notified by phone. It is okay to outsource this task to your support person. It can also be healing to make the calls yourself, if you are ready. These people will most likely be additional sources of moral support. You can also share funeral arrangements at this time. Once all family and close friends have been informed, it is fine to post the news to social media. You might also choose to place an obituary in the local newspaper (the funeral home will help with this).

Notify Your Employer and Your Loved One's Employer

If your loved one was employed, notify the employer after you've called family. If you don't know who to speak with, ask for someone in the human resources department. If you are employed, it's likely you used up all or most of your paid time off (PTO) caring for your loved one. But you also need time to plan and attend the funeral, as well as time to grieve. Most employers will extend courtesy time and even offer to help however they can. Contact your employer immediately. Don't feel forced to share details if you are not ready to speak about it. A simple notification is sufficient: "I had a death in my family. My (relative) passed away, and I need X days off for the funeral and grieving. Please forgive me—I'm not ready to share details." Ask your boss to share the news with your coworkers, if you are comfortable with that. You need support, and your coworkers could be helpful. Respectfully request that coworkers do not share the news on social media. You should be in control of when and where to post it.

Acquire the Death Certificate

A death certificate is legally required to be issued when a death occurs and will be necessary as you make funeral arrangements and take care of personal, financial, and legal business on behalf of the person who died and his or her estate. The physician or medical examiner validates the death, and a licensed funeral director confirms the proper handling of the body. The funeral director will file it with the county health department within seventy-two hours. Be aware of how many copies of the death certificate you're going to need. You'll need copies when notifying most financial accounts, including life insurance companies, Social Security, and VA accounts, and a copy for filing the final tax return. But you can't just photocopy them. They need to be official. The recommended number of official copies is ten, at about $10–$12 apiece.

Look for Important Paperwork

Important paperwork includes everything from life insurance policies to bank account statements to bills and subscriptions, as well as Internet passwords. Look for it sooner rather than later so that you are prepared. Following are a few specifics you'll want to consider:

- Life insurance companies receive notice of a death without you having to inform them. You may want to call them to be certain, but if you are a beneficiary on the policy, you will likely receive the check in time to help cover funeral costs and outstanding bills.

- Bank accounts should be closed within the first month, after all automatic withdrawals have been identified and canceled. Some accounts incur monthly fees if the balance goes below a certain amount. If you discover an open account eight months down the road, call the bank to negotiate fee reimbursement.

- If a last will and testament is involved, reach out to the lawyer who prepared the document. His or her name should be on the paperwork.

- Contact Social Security and Medicare.

- Pay bills and cancel subscriptions, credit cards, and monthly services (such as gardeners or housecleaners).

- Get access to the safe-deposit box or home safe.

- Find passwords and usernames to access online accounts.

- Forward email to yourself for a few months to make sure you've taken care of all business before closing email and social media accounts.

- Deal with property and income taxes. If property taxes have not been paid in a while, a home could be subject to foreclosure. If you can't find the paperwork, you might be able to look it up online through the county tax assessor's office. If your loved one worked with a tax accountant, call him or her to schedule an appointment.

Be aware that all online accounts, including email and social media sites, have terms of service that we agree to when we create the account. If you do not have access to usernames and passwords, and you don't have power of attorney, you will likely have to go through a lengthy process to close the accounts.

I'm no stranger to death. Despite providing the best treatment available, someone inevitably dies in my ICU almost every day. I am no longer shocked to learn that families have no idea how to proceed, and I believe that what I say or do in response matters. I know that dying is a part of living, and so I try to open the conversation regarding the spiritual and practical—funeral arrangements and legal documents—in an effort to guide family members when they are facing this situation. But in an emotional state, families only hear so much. And so my plea to you is to move through any resistance that may be holding you back and take the time to prepare for your own passing, if only for the sake of your loved ones.

ACTION Take Time to Reflect

As you're sorting through documents and making phone calls, many memories are likely to surface. Take some time to remember good times with your loved one. Jot them down in a notebook or journal.

Caring for You

Don't be too hard on yourself by wishing you'd done or said something earlier so that last wishes and arrangements would have been more organized. There's only so much you can do. What's done is done. Move forward and make a point not to judge yourself or anyone else but to make the best of the circumstances.

Main Chapter Takeaways

- Many people do not know what steps to take after a loved one dies, and not everyone is emotionally prepared to take next steps.

- Helping families through the process is healing for everyone involved.

- Asking for support—whether from the medical team or a family member or friend—is always the first step.

- When last wishes aren't known, gather family and friends to talk about how to proceed with funeral arrangements.

- When last wishes are known, ask others to help you with the arrangements.

- Finding important documents, closing accounts, and tending to other details can be more work than you expect—ask for help.

Planning an Event You
Don't Want to Attend

One of my wealthiest patients was cofounder of a bakery empire and a cooking-channel star. He was a smart man. At the age of ninety-two, as he lay in the ICU with an infection and in multi-organ failure, his son was left to unwind the intricacies of his life. Though he was close to his son, this man was so private that it took a court order and a police escort to gain access to his house, as well as months to locate his bank accounts, safe-deposit boxes, and will. All the while, he lingered in a terrible state while his son was filled with anguish, unsure about what to do. This man's choices had a ripple effect on how his loving family and medical team were able to care for him.

How many times have I seen similar situations? As a physician who works with end-stage lung disease—more times than I care to count. Wealthy people are as guilty as those without much to pass on. Music icon Prince is a prime example. Prince died in 2016 of an opioid overdose without a will, placing his $200 million estate in the hands of Minnesota courts. A year after his passing, the estate was still tied up in court, and disputes among potential heirs had escalated. We'll never know why Prince didn't create a will. But most of us might admit that we can understand. I personally don't know anyone who gets excited about planning for the time when they will die. I usually talk about it in terms of planning an event we don't want to attend. But when we put it in perspective, planning for this inevitability makes the best of sense. It's the kindest thing we can do. Yet most of us resist. We put it on the back burner. Even the thought of researching advance directives and estate planning and then filling out a flood of forms that we'll likely have to update every year or so is off-putting. What's the incentive, really, in preparing for a day most of us don't look forward to, much less think about?

Allow me to ask a few thought-provoking (hopefully) questions: Who wants to be a burden in their old age? Wouldn't you prefer that the house were clutter-free, inheritance plans laid out, debts paid, and all-important documents signed and dated? Wouldn't you also want your family to know and honor your wishes? Maybe you've at least thought about what you want for a send-off, whether a traditional funeral, your ashes dispersed over the Himalayas, or the party of the century. Giving this some forethought is a pretty good deal, really. You get what you want, and your family is not left grappling with difficult medical decisions, tearing the house apart searching for documents, or spending what would have been their inheritance on lawyers and court fees. Intellectually, we know this is true. So why do more than half of Americans put off these preparations and conversations until it's too late?

Some of it might have to do with awareness. According to a German study, a large percentage of people aren't aware that health-care proxies are even a thing. The researchers surveyed a group of cancer patients and a group of healthy controls, as well as physicians and nursing staff, questioning them about advance directives. Surprisingly, only 10 percent of the medical staff had advance directives in place, compared to almost twice as many patients and healthy controls (18 and 19 percent, respectively). But a majority of participants had good intentions: 50 to 81 percent had it on their wish list of things to do. The cancer patients were at the high end of the range. Not counting the medical staff, only 36 percent of participants knew that they could appoint a health-care agent. Among all three groups, about half thought that family members could abuse such documents.[1]

So clearly, trust can be an issue when it comes to advance directives. And perhaps uncertainty—how do we know how we'll feel about our plans when the time comes? Some patients tell me that they don't understand the procedures well enough to make these types of decisions. And what about the gray areas? All of this can add up to failure to take action. But I believe there's more to it than lack of knowledge or understanding. My patients tell me that talking about or planning for their death makes it "real" and that the thought of dying provokes anxiety.

Start with Baby Steps

If lack of understanding is keeping you from completing advance directives, start by getting the information you need. Many insurance providers will pay for advance directive sessions with a clinician if done during a wellness exam. Medicare started covering the cost in 2016.

I like to suggest that people schedule an appointment with their family doctor, review the documents, and ask questions such as these:

- What is involved with each of these procedures (intubation, resuscitation) and why would I choose not to do them?
- What happens if I have a chance at recovery? Where do doctors draw the line?
- How can I trust that the doctor treating me will follow my orders?
- How can I trust that my family will follow my orders?
- How do I ensure that the hospital knows about my directives? What if something happens to me while traveling out of the country, for instance? Or out of the state?
- Can my health-care agent go against my directives?
- My wife knows what I want. Can't she just make the decision for me?

If you're not ready to fill out the paperwork after the session, take it home with you and process what you learned. Talk to close family members about what they think. Consider who might make a good health-care agent. But mark a date on your calendar for when you will decide what to do and make sure to follow through; otherwise, the task becomes a moving target. I've been guilty of postponing the updates on my own will. You just have to make it a priority and get it done.

Anxiety: The Only Reaction Available

For some people, preparing for the day they will die provokes a low level of anxiety. For others, it creates an exaggerated emotional response. In the field of psychology, this response is known as "death anxiety," which some people experience as dread or fear whenever they think of dying.

Death anxiety is a fairly recent cultural phenomenon. Anxiety, for instance, is never mentioned in any of the historical descriptions of the dying process. Plenty of studies argue that before the 1800s, conversations about death and dying occurred more naturally and regularly than they do today. People used to talk about death and prepare themselves and their family. But tremendous advances in medicine have given people the perception that we are invincible. We do not go into old age or terminal illness having had this conversation about death and dying and forgiveness. When that conversation has not taken place, the only human reaction available to us is anxiety and frustration.

Where Do You Stand?

Anxiety over death and dying is the most common emotion I see in the ICU. I see this over and over again, so much so that I mentally categorize families into groups based on their emotional response to death. One group—a very small number of families—react to the news of an impending death with little or no anxiety. They hold a mature understanding that life is finite. They sit calmly with their loved one and are fully present with the death experience. They don't like it, but they have accepted it, and so they don't fight it. These people have come to terms with the fact that their loved one will soon pass. They understand life, and so they understand death.

I remember vividly my first on-call shift at the Cleveland Clinic. I tended to the family of a patient who was actively dying of multiple complications from cancer. He was fully conscious, with two daughters and his wife at his bedside. They seemed to me to truly comprehend life's limitations. They were sad, but no one was screaming or yelling.

They understood that he was about to die. To this day—many years afterward—this family remains an example to many in the ICU. And it started with the patient. Full of disease and shortness of breath, he never showed any signs of anxiety. Even when he had little strength left, he would muster a smile when I walked into the room and asked a question. That to me is the real treatment for any level of death anxiety—the real treatment does not come in a pill but stems from accepting that death is a part of life.

The second group, which is the majority of families, displays tremendous anxiety. They scream, holler, blame, and fight. I believe that what they are really fighting is not each other but the idea of death because they have not accepted death as being a part of life. I suspect that they have never made any effort to think about death much less talk about it. Surprisingly, I find that many medical professionals fall into this group.

At one point in my career, I was called in to intervene with a family that was being particularly difficult. The patient was an eighty-nine-year-old mom suffering from heart failure, advanced diabetes, terminal gastric cancer, and chronic pain. Her family consisted of three practicing physicians. One of them was also a professor at a respected university. These siblings were blessed with drive, intelligence, and a great deal of compassion for their mother. They were also plagued with anxiety. How do I know? As soon as they entered the ICU, these otherwise rational scientists became the most irrational people on the planet.

I'm not exaggerating when I say that every single day they were fighting with everybody within range—firing nurses, firing doctors, demanding their mother receive more attention. The dissonance led to one battle after another. They "fired" a nurse for not giving medications right on time and berated an intern for not knowing the exact value of a blood test. Housekeeping, which did an amazing job keeping the area spotless and sterile, walked on eggshells when they passed her room. They'd been reprimanded by this family multiple times. The siblings also bickered among themselves about which treatments were most appropriate, including whether to perform a tracheostomy and insert a feeding tube. The family's outbursts were out of line and adversely affecting their mother's care. No one wanted to enter the room when the clan was present. It felt like the Hatfields *and* McCoys together against the treatment team.

I was in charge of critical care at the time and was called in toward the end to see if I could somehow calm their fury. I must say I was somewhat intimidated. Others had tried and been cast aside. It can be hard to rationalize with rage of this magnitude—what words could possibly quell a raging sea?

The only thing that I asked was that we all be in a room together. I felt it was important to see their facial expressions, body language, and emotional reactions. And I wanted to address each of them individually. I consider nonverbal communication the highway to compassionate care. They quickly agreed. Although they lived in different cities, all three of them were staying in the area to keep watch over their mom's condition. The four of us sat down at a table in a hospital conference room.

"How can I help you navigate these waters?" I started. I let them talk, and by the middle of the conversation, I realized that they were not talking with each other. I don't know if they even heard each other. They were in overdrive, unable to stop their chatter, feeling that only their words counted. After ten minutes of this, I interrupted. "You know what, how can we do the very best for your mom, given the circumstances that she is in today? Without blaming anyone, how can we fix this? How can we fix it and get the best outcome?"

My words did nothing, and their accusations grew bigger and more pronounced. So I resorted to what I know best. "Let me stop you right there," I insisted. "I'm going to tell you one truth. One day, your mom is going to be gone from this planet. I'm convinced—I'm 100 percent convinced—that there is not a single parent out there who doesn't want their children to be united in these kinds of situations. I'm convinced. What do you guys think?"

The daughter broke out crying, "I've been having this feeling that we have been interfering with her care because we know medicine, and we have forgotten that we are humans, that she is human."

My words were simple, but they resonated with the siblings. The focus went from the anxiety of having the medical knowledge but not the ability to save their dying mother to patient-centered care. To each of them, her death meant failure. So they, more than most, fell prey to the misguided belief that modern medicine always has an answer. Much to everyone's relief, during the five weeks their mother remained in the hospital, the focus moved from them to her. This transition not only took the pressure off of these talented clinicians, but allowed the family to feel what anxiety so cleverly disguises: love, compassion, and presence of mind.

The third group of families falls somewhere in-between. A balance of acceptance and anxiety leaves them in control but visibly upset. They may lash out at staff, but their behavior isn't outrageous. They settle down eventually, but not without displaying signs of anxiety, including blaming, distrusting, and even sulking.

Neither socioeconomic status nor education nor age plays a role in determining which group a family falls into. My belief is that the more we've allowed ourselves to talk about death and to treat it as a part of life, the more naturally we will respond to the inevitability of it. I have seen this in even the most traumatic of cases.

Matt was a charming college student who was about to finish all his premed class requirements when he was hit by a drunk driver. He was taken to the ICU where I was working. He suffered multiple injuries, including major head trauma and rib fractures. I met his father and mother soon after he was transferred from the operating room to the ICU. They were anxious, crying, and in total disbelief. Dr. Thompson, the neurosurgeon, came to meet them while we were talking. He explained in detail the severity of the brain damage and the procedure he had performed to help decrease the intracranial pressure. The more he talked, the more confused the parents became. All of a sudden, the mom interrupted, "Will he survive? Is he brain dead?"

"I don't know, Ma'am. Time will tell," Dr. Thompson replied.

During the next four days, I saw a parade of family, friends, college students, and neighbors coming and going. Matt remained unconscious. On day five, he was pronounced brain dead. I came back to work on day six and witnessed his mother, father, and siblings painfully saying good-bye to Matt. They hugged each other and cried and prayed around his bed. Later I passed by Matt's room again and ran into his father. He was thanking the medical team for everything. I could sense the pain in his heart when he told me, "Unexpected, for sure. . . . I wish I could stop time, but I can't. This is life."

Preparation Relieves Anxiety

Dr. L. Nelson Bell, a medical missionary and the father-in-law of famous evangelist Billy Graham, once said, "Only those who are prepared to die are really prepared to live."[2] I'm going to take his statement literally.

Death is such a mystery. It has colonized our awareness, but the fear of death dominates how we respond. We don't recognize that we are born to die and that it's a reality that will happen whether we reject it or not. And so we are prone to put off anything that has to do with death and dying. It's our way of resisting what we don't want to face. History tells us that when we are prepared to die, our lives are actually better. Thinking about end-of-life choices can improve the quality of life now and toward the end. Even more important, it eases the burden on family. So expressing our wishes should be one of our most important priorities. "Only those who are prepared to die are really prepared to live."

The experiences people go through after the death of a loved one can sometimes motivate them to get their own affairs in order. I saw this with one of my patient's brothers. During his sister's last day, he endured his nephews fighting over everything. Within weeks, he had prepared a trust with all of his wishes clearly stated. We might be encouraged to model the steps of someone we know. But if things didn't go smoothly, we can also learn from another's mistakes.

Start When You Move Out of Your Parents' Home

Planning for our dying day is important at any age. In the same week in the ICU, I treated a nineteen-year-old man and a fifty-year-old woman. The woman, Caroline, had been married to her husband for five years before they had separated for about twenty-five years. But they had never officially divorced. For the past ten years, she had been living with and sharing her life with her boyfriend, Bob. One day, Caroline's blood pressure suddenly spiked, and she suffered a stroke. She wound up in a hospital bed in a persistent vegetative state. Her prognosis was dim. Recovery from a massive intracranial bleed is very unlikely. Caroline's legal husband, we learned through talking with Bob, had died five years earlier. Bob was crying and confused. The case manager reached out to the hospital's legal department to find ways to help him, but their hands were tied because Caroline had never given Bob power of attorney. And then her children, who had not been a part of her life for a very long time, arrived from out of state. Meanwhile, Bob was dealing with the emotions of being unable to help Caroline. She needed to be moved to an LTAC facility, but the health insurance company was asking for a financial report, and no one had access to Caroline's accounts. This story is happening in my ICU as I write this chapter. Imagine all of the complications still to come. We are right there taking care of Caroline and listening to Bob's frustrations and concerns daily.

At the same time, I have a nineteen-year-old named Jake who went to a party and was found in the early hours of the next morning on the street. Someone had brutally assaulted him, resulting in him being brain dead but still functioning in the ICU. His girlfriend, Linda, showed up at the hospital. Linda said with complete confidence that he had expressed to her that he didn't want to remain on a machine. His parents, however, did not know about his wishes. This has created a major division. At nineteen, Jake is an adult capable of making his own medical decisions, yet in the absence of a written document, determining who is the most suited to making that decision for him can be difficult. In this case, the ethics committee got involved, and his parents and girlfriend agreed to work together without involving the court system.

I strongly believe that when children leave their parents' home or are living independently, they should have written end-of-life wishes and express them clearly. We live in an age with access to thousands of apps that help us find coffee shops and trivial facts, but no one seems to know where to turn to make these important plans. We all need this. It is imperative to society.

I'm hoping these stories (and perhaps stories you've heard from others) will give you the perspective you need to move beyond any anxiety you might have. But what if you need to broach this sensitive topic with a family member? I'd like to share some stories of how some people have successfully handled this.

Asking the Delicate Questions

After hearing me speak on the subject of advance directives, Stacy, one of my newer physician assistants, approached me. She told me that hearing my speeches and working in the ICU had opened her eyes to how important preparing for death is and that she had never thought about it before. Stacy is from a blended family with six siblings who are all incredibly close, yet the subject of death and dying has never come up. The family is strong financially and owns several properties. Stacy asked me how she could approach the subject with her parents. She felt that bringing it up out of the blue would seem odd. She didn't want her parents to think she was asking for the wrong reasons.

My advice was to use the passing of someone close to the family to bring up the subject: "Mom, Helen had a very nice, traditional funeral. I think I would rather be cremated. What do you think you would want?" Or discuss advance directives with your doctor at your annual exam and mention it to Dad: "Yesterday, at my wellness exam, I filled out a health-care proxy and a living will. I made you my health-care agent. I feel really good about taking care of this. I think you should think about doing this too." The small amount of time it takes to pass on subtle comments can be highly effective.

Here's what Stacy did: She went around trying to convince her siblings of the need for this conversation with their parents, but they were resistant. Since she wasn't able to persuade them, she took a backdoor approach. She and three of her sisters belong to the same book club. The next time it was her turn to pick the book, Stacy chose *Being Mortal* by Atul Gawande. They read the book together over the course of a month, and by the end of the month, the sisters were on board. The women developed a plan for how to approach their parents. The next time the family had dinner together, they would bring up the book they read at book club and then ask some very specific questions. At the family dinner table, conversation was usually pretty lively, so they felt their parents would chime in.

"Where would you want to die? In a hospital or at home?" Stacy started. Mom and Dad both responded that they didn't want to die at the hospital. The next question was if you don't want to die at the hospital, how will the medical team know? Stacy explained that if one of them fell terminally ill today, at this moment, the family would call 911, and they would be taken to die in the hospital, unless they had specified otherwise in an advance directive. The parents were not aware that they could take these steps.

The first few questions in the conversation were hard, very hard, for Stacy. But her parents quickly accepted the logic behind doing some planning and how it could curb anxiety for everyone involved. Stacy was pretty clever.

One of my aunts, who was very close to everyone in the family, was dying of pancreatic cancer here in Miami. She was separated geographically from her two children: her older son is a neurosurgeon in Spain, and her other son was living in Cuba. Her husband had passed two years earlier. Her sons contacted me with questions about treating the cancer. Advanced pancreatic cancer is difficult to treat, and the survival rate posttreatment is low. Her sons were afraid she would not understand that filling out advance directives was important now, so I agreed to talk to her.

I sat with her and I said, "Listen, I haven't mentioned this before because we Cubans are really afraid of cancer, but one day I'm going to die—we all are going to die. But if I die today or you die today, it is important that we express our wishes to our family, so they understand what to do and what not to do. We are living in a time when they will call an ambulance, and they will take you to the hospital. In the absence of any document expressing your desires and your feelings, the medical team is going to do everything they can to keep you alive, but in the end, it will produce a lot of pain and still not help in the long run. Inevitably, we are all going to die."

My aunt understood, and she completed the paperwork. We followed this up with a phone conversation with her sons. We recorded the conversation, and it was the most beautiful thing. She said she wanted to have a photograph made of the entire extended family. Her son flew in from Spain to be with her. *Beautiful.*

Bear in mind that a lot of older adults are unaware of the medical procedures that are available to us to support life. They also remember the days when you called the family doctor, who made a house call. Today you call 911, and an ambulance takes you to the hospital. This single change has tripped up more people than you might realize. This is why I strongly believe in informing older adults about what is going to happen in the long run. Most people want to die at home, but they end up in the hospital.

"I'm Not a Planner!"

Some people are planners and others aren't. It's true we can't plan for everything. Life happens. But death is inevitable. We know it will happen; we just don't know when. If we're unconscious, we won't have a say in what happens to us. So really we're taking a gamble. But last-minute planning is an option for those who suddenly find themselves with a serious illness and with their faculties intact.

Just the day before yesterday, I was called in to see a patient, Jack. He had gone to the emergency room complaining of neck pain, and when they did a CT scan, they saw a mass on his neck. When they did a CT scan of his chest, it revealed a mass in his lungs. A two-pack-a-day smoker for more than forty years, Jack was now likely suffering from lung cancer and cervical metastasis—the cancer had spread from his lungs to his spine in his neck. This man had no other symptoms, just some neck pain, and suddenly he was facing this devastating reality.

Jack was a very well-known contractor. He was very good at what he did and was wealthy as a result. He didn't get that way by being unorganized, but Jack could never have prepared for that moment of truth in the hospital. I came into his room to examine his lungs, and he asked me what I thought his prognosis was. I told him I didn't know and that nobody really knows. I've seen a patient with advanced lung cancer survive more than ten years despite the odds. I then added that I do know one thing: whether this is the event or not, you need to prepare. Jack was a big guy, over six feet tall, and kind of tough looking, so I was surprised when he started to cry. He admitted he was scared—scared of dying, scared of having cancer, and scared because he hadn't planned anything.

The next day, I came in, and he was calling his lawyer to prepare a trust. He had started going through the process. At that moment, I felt a tremendous success. Even if cancer takes his life, Jack will be able to get his affairs in order.

Today, most doctors' offices have access to advance directives. Or you can Google "advance directives" and find a website that will not only give you guidance regarding advance directives but simple steps you can take to help put your finances in order. Unless you have a lot of assets, you don't have to see a lawyer to create a legally binding document. If you have access to a lawyer, that's great. But most people can start with a simple approach.

Last Will and Testament: Tips for "Keeping the Peace"

Most squabbles over family heirlooms and property happen because of lack of communication and false expectations—expectations people assume and keep to themselves. Often, expectations are based on what people feel they deserve. Grown children sometimes see a possession passed down as a display of love—love they deserve. Communicating your wishes can put an end to false expectations and help avoid conflict. When you throw in some of the values you'd like to pass on, family members are less likely to battle it out for possessions. If your family is a complex web of step-brothers and step-sisters, significant others, or siblings who don't get along, it's even more important to specify your wishes.

Some of us may have only a few things to wrap up—maybe sign a quitclaim deed (a legal document issued to transfer interest in real property) and ensure that our loved ones know we have a life insurance policy to cover the cost of a funeral. Maybe we want all the kids to know that Jessica gets the diamond wedding ring and Elliot gets the car. These details can be important. Even if this knowledge sits with the kids for twenty years, they know what to expect. If you have to sell the diamond ring and the car before you pass, so be it. Make that clear too. ᔤ

Getting Comfortable with the Idea

If I had things my way, planning for our own death would be as commonplace and as easy to do as sharing what kind of birthday cake we want on our special day. But I would say that it will take time for us as a society to feel that way. Likely, the acceptance of death and dying will always be a big issue for all of us, but that doesn't mean that we shouldn't plan and make our wishes clear.

In my opinion, end-of-life education should be crafted into high school and college curricula. I believe in embracing every aspect of education to increase the conversation regarding this topic, and I hope we start seeing better outreach.

In *The 7 Habits of Highly Effective People*, Stephen Covey suggests a visualization exercise as a way to reflect on character. Basically, we are supposed to imagine our funeral and listen to what people have to say about us. I am hoping that people will talk about me as a loving father and husband and a compassionate caregiver. I will take it a step further and add what I do not want: I do not want people complaining that I left my affairs in disarray, creating mayhem and discord among my family.

I wasn't at Prince's funeral, but I imagine that, for some people, the shock of not having a will turned the conversation from all the good he'd managed to do in his life to "What was he thinking?" And so I ask: How do you want your family to remember you? What will your legacy be? If given the opportunity, would you choose a graceful exit?

ACTION   Visualize Your Funeral

In the mode of Stephen Covey, visualize your funeral—not so much to imagine what others might say about you, but to see what type of event it is that you're choosing.

Caring for You

Embrace resistance. In *The War of Art*, author Steven Pressfield explains that resistance is a sign that we are not doing something we really *should* be doing. Resistance is the ego fighting the spirit's will. His solution is to sit down and do what you're resisting, whether it be writing, painting, or filling out forms.

Main Chapter Takeaways

- Planning for our death helps ensure our last wishes are met and minimizes stress among family members.

- Most of us put these plans on the back burner.

- Medicare and other insurances now cover end-of-life care planning discussions with a doctor during a wellness exam.

- Get answers to your questions about advance directives.

- Most of us harbor some level of death anxiety. Preparation relieves anxiety.

- It's never too early to begin planning.

- Encourage others to do the same.

For Every Season

When I was in my teens, one of my uncles, along with his entire family, died in a car accident. I remember vividly the day my father got the phone call. On the other end of the line, a voice told him that my uncle and his family had been heading out of our hometown when their vehicle was crushed by a truck. The whole family, all four of them, died instantly. The tragedy had a profound effect on my parents. It reopened a wound in my mom's heart, a wound left by the death of her first son, who was only eleven months old when he died. The fear of losing another child became the focus of her life, and she was tossed into a valley of depression that lasted years. My dad and grandma suffered in silence. All kinds of fears marked those years, but at the core was the fear of death.

The tragic accident changed them, but it didn't seem to change me, at least not profoundly. I was a teenager looking at life through my own little prism, and I just thought that life was going to go on. I imagine that if the accident had involved my parents or a sibling, I would have been much more distraught. But to this day, what I remember most about that event are my cousins and how we used to play on my father's farm during the summertime. I don't focus on the horror of it all. I am somehow able to retain my adolescent viewpoint: death, even when accidental, is natural.

Somewhere along the way, as we mature and go through life's seasons, facing life's many ups and downs, we lose sight of how natural death is. We turn our focus to how the loss affects us personally. We grow fearful of death because we equate it with loss: one more disappointment, one more person to miss, one person fewer in our corner.

The death of a loved one has the potential to bring us full circle, to bring us back to the state of mind of our more spiritual, youthful self, when death, even tragic accidents, seemed normal. And then to take us further yet, to a place only those in the summer, fall, or winter of life can fully comprehend, until we reach the place where we look at death not through the prism of how it adversely changes our personal life but how it changes us personally. Death finally brings us to the core of our humanity, where we need to answer those universal questions, the ones boiling in every human's heart, the questions of existence, purpose, and destiny.

For me, as I witness death and feel the loss of those around me nearly every day, I become more and more committed to living with intention. I tell my kids over and over that we need to aspire to minimize fear and regret at the end of life by living in the present—being intentional and enjoying each day to the fullest. Every time a loved one comes to mind, I text or call them. I have been doing this for the last six or seven years. I do not let those moments pass by. And it feels wonderful. I want to do this until my last breath. I want my life to run the course planned by God to the fullest—from beginning to end. I don't know what's going to happen. I could be in a car accident today or tomorrow, so I try to grab those precious moments that can truly build memories and that I imagine are part of fulfilling my life's purpose.

People we love and who love us need to hear over and over that we love them, that we trust them, and that we value them. This is something that everyone silently asks of all the people around them—show me that you care, that you love me unconditionally, that you are quick to forgive me, and that you will not judge me. These are pearls of wisdom I've learned from my parents and my patients.

Death shows us how finite and fragile life is on this earth. When we accept that death is inevitable for ourselves, living with intention and in the present becomes far easier. We're not unconsciously preoccupied with resentments and fears. We're able to open up to the life before us and make the most of it now. When we do this, conditions are ripe for a full, authentic life, as well as for our own graceful exit.

No regrets, no fears, no chaos.

Just love.

Acknowledgments

In writing this book I have been blessed with a wonderful team. At the top of the list I want to thank Liz Neporent, who first saw the potential of this book and quickly introduced me to Linda Konner. A big thanks to Linda Konner, my wonderful agent, who introduced me to Sounds True.

I especially want to thank Karen Chernyaev for her excellent writing skills. I enjoyed working with you as this book gradually took shape.

My sincerest thanks also to the following people:

Caroline Pincus, my Sounds True editor, for your insight and guidance.

My administrative team, Samantha Feola and Loren Pizarro, for your support of this vision.

Lisa Tener, who guided me in other projects and introduced me to the Harvard Writer's Conference, where I met Liz and Linda.

US Army Major General (Ret.) Bernard Loeffke, an American hero, medical missionary, author, and speaker. Thank you for your advice and comments on the book proposal.

My medical team, Dr. Monica Egozcue, Dr. Hector Vazquez, Fanny Tsi, and Tara Rowland. Thanks for your hard work.

My parents, Miguelina (Grandma Lina) and Domingo (Grandpa Guito), for giving me life and the best family on the planet. Mom, your energy is contagious and "love" gains meaning in you. Thank you for the morning *cafecitos*.

My brother, Yoel, and sister-in-law, Bertha, for your love and support.

Burke Lennihan, a gifted writer. I appreciate your insight.

To the love of my life, Nicole, for always believing in me. I will say it again and again—I'm convinced God opened the floodgates of heaven and blessed me the day I met you. You are the cornerstone of my family. I love you more and more.

My beloved children, my life would be incomplete without you. You continue to bring joy and love to my life. I'm constantly learning from you. I'm so proud of each of you. Diego's determination to change the world continues to inspire me; Amanda's knowledge, love, and compassion encourage me; Lauren, a gifted writer, your determination and optimism motivate me. I see great leaders in each of you. I thank God for the privilege of being called your daddy!

Above all, I want to thank my Lord Jesus Christ for rescuing me.

Gustavo Ferrer, MD

Notes

Chapter 1: Getting Everyone on the Same Page

1. David W. Molloy, Roger M. Clarnette, E. Ann Braun, Martin R. Eisemann, and B. Sneiderman, "Decision Making in the Incompetent Elderly: 'The Daughter from California Syndrome,'" *Journal of the American Geriatrics Society* 39, no. 4 (April 1991): 396–399, dx.doi.org/10.1111/j.1532-5415.1991.tb02907.x.

2. Jaya K. Rao, Lynda A. Anderson, Feng-Chang Lin, and Jeffrey P. Laux, "Completion of Advance Directives among U.S. Consumers," *American Journal of Preventive Medicine* 46, no. 1 (January 2014): 65–70, dx.doi.org/10.1016/j.amepre.2013.09.008.

Chapter 2: Letting Head and Heart Guide You Through the Hardest Decisions

1. National Hospice and Palliative Care Organization, *NHPCO Facts and Figures: Hospice Care in America* (2016), 5, nhpco.org/sites/default/files/public/Statistics_Research/2016_Facts_Figures.pdf.

Chapter 3: Your Best Ally

1. William G. Finn and E. Blair Holladay, "Discordant Interpretations of Breast Biopsy Specimens by Pathologists," *Journal of the American Medical Association* 314, no. 1 (July 2015): 82, dx.doi.org/10.1001/jama.2015.6230.

Chapter 4: What to Do When Your Loved One Still Has Some Time

1. Chi Chan Lee, Osman Perez, Alwiya Saleh, Armando Cabrera, Nillian Zamot, Mauricio Danckers, and Gustavo Ferrer, "Families Perception, Knowledge, and Psychological Stress of Transitions of Care From the ICU: Improving Transition of Care," *CHEST* 152, no. 4, supplement (October 2017): A560, dx.doi.org/10.1016/j.chest.2017.08.590.

2. Loraine A. West, Samantha Cole, Daniel Goodkind, and Wan He, *65+ in the United States: 2010,* U.S. Census Bureau (June 2014), 50, census.gov/content/dam/Census/library/publications/2014/demo/p23-212.pdf.

Chapter 5: Who Pays?

1. Berhanu Alemayehu and Kenneth E. Warner, "The Lifetime Distribution of Health Care Costs," *Health Services Research* 39, no. 3 (June 2004): 627–642, dx.doi.org/10.1111/j.1475-6773.2004.00248.x.

2. Samuel Marshall, Kathleen McGarry, and Jonathan Skinner, "The Risk of Out-of-Pocket Health Care Expenditure at End of Life (Working Paper 16170)," National Bureau of Economic Research Working Paper Series (July 2010), dx.doi.org/10.3386/w16170.

3. MetLife Mature Market Institute, *Market Survey of Long-Term Care Costs: The 2012 MetLife Market Survey of Nursing Home, Assisted Living, Adult Day Services, and Home Care Costs* (November 2012), 5, metlife.com/assets/cao/mmi/publications/studies/2012/studies/mmi-2012-market-survey-long-term-care-costs.pdf.

4. Jennifer M. Ortman, Victoria A. Velkoff, and Howard Hogan, *An Aging Nation: The Older Population in the United States; Population Estimates and Projections, Current Population Reports,* U.S. Census Bureau (May 2014), 6, census.gov/prod/2014pubs/p25-1140.pdf.

5. "Life Expectancy in the USA, 1900–98: Men and Women," (n.d.), accessed October 18, 2016, u.demog.berkeley. edu/~andrew/1918/figure2.html.

Chapter 6: Legacies and Regrets

1. William Osler, *The Principles and Practice of Medicine: Designed for the Use of Practitioners and Students of Medicine* (New York and London: D. Appleton and Company, 1921), 79, archive.org/stream/principlesandpr00mccrgoog#page/n106/mode/2up/search/friend+of+the+aged.
2. Elizabeth Fine, M. Carrington Reid, Rouzi Shengelia, and Ronald D. Adelman, "Directly Observed Patient–Physician Discussions in Palliative and End-of-Life Care: A Systematic Review of the Literature," *Journal of Palliative Medicine* 13, no. 5 (May 2010): 595–603, dx.doi.org/10.1089/jpm.2009.0388.

Chapter 7: Grieving, Letting Go, and Acceptance

1. Carlos Fernández de Larrea et al., "Childhood Tuberculosis in the Warao Population in Venezuela," *Investigación Clínica* 43, no. 1 (2002): 35–48.
2. Julian A. Villalba et al., "Low Child Survival Index in a Multi-Dimensionally Poor Amerindian Population in Venezuela," *PLOS ONE* (December 2013), dx.doi.org/10.1371/journal.pone.0085638.

Chapter 8: Post-Death Paperwork

1. Margaret I. Fitch, Tracey DasGupta, and Bill Ford, "Achieving Excellence in Palliative Care: Perspectives of Health Care Professionals," *Asia-Pacific Journal of Oncology Nursing* 3, no. 1 (March 2016): 66–72, dx.doi.org/10.4103/2347-5625.164999; Anette Fosse, Sabine Ruths, Kirsti Malterud, and Margrethe Aase Schaufel, "Doctors' Learning Experiences in End-of-Life Care—A Focus Group Study from Nursing Homes," *BMC Medical Education* 27, no. 17 (January 2017): dx.doi.org/10.1186/s12909-017-0865-8.

Chapter 9: Planning an Event You Don't Want to Attend

1. S. Sahm, R. Will, and G. Hommel, "Attitudes Towards and Barriers to Writing Advance Directives Amongst Cancer Patients, Healthy Controls, and Medical Staff," *Journal of Medical Ethics* 31, no. 8 (August 2005): 437–440, dx.doi. org/10.1136/jme.2004.009605.
2. L. Nelson Bell, quoted in Billy Graham, *Death and the Life After* (Nashville, TN: W Publishing Group, 1987), 4.

About the Author

Gustavo Ferrer, MD, is pulmonologist trained in Cuba and the United States, founder of the Cleveland Clinic Florida's Chronic Cough Clinic, and president of Intensive Care Experts based in south Florida. An authority on respiratory ailments with more than twenty years' experience, Dr. Ferrer grew up in a culture that effectively uses herbal teas and folk remedies for relief from various afflictions, and today his work encompasses both traditional and modern forms of medicine. Dr. Ferrer grew up in a remote, rural area of Cuba, where he learned compassionate care from his mother and grandmother. As director of Respiratory Research for the United Nations University in Venezuela, he witnessed how one of the oldest tribes in South America handled death and dying. In 2000, he came to the United States and retrained with a residency in Texas and a pulmonary and critical care fellowship at George Washington University in Washington, DC. He then joined the Cleveland Clinic Florida. He has delivered more than three hundred presentations at local, national, and international medical meetings and is currently involved in multiple research studies. In 2011, Dr. Ferrer was appointed to the prestigious National Steering Committee for the COPD Alliance. As part of this esteemed group, he attended a White House briefing to discuss the Affordable Care Act. He has since received several prestigious awards, including Best Doctors in the US by *U.S. News & World Report*, Most Compassionate Doctor, Patients' Choice Award, and multiple teaching awards. Dr. Ferrer has been featured in *USA Today* and the *Miami Herald* and on NBC News, CNN en Español, and Radio Caracol in Miami. He has also been featured in many Latin American national newspapers. He is the author of *Cough Cures: The Complete Guide to the Best Natural*

Remedies and Over-the-Counter Drugs for Acute and Chronic Coughs and *Cura Tu Tos con los Remedios de Abuelita.* Dr. Ferrer also created a series of continuing-education lectures and training materials that focus on dealing with end-stage diseases. This material teaches physicians, nurses, and other medical professionals how to support the families of terminally ill patients with kindness and compassion. He is continually striving to improve health care in America. He can be contacted at gustavoferrermd.com.

About Sounds True

Sounds True is a multimedia publisher whose mission is to inspire and support personal transformation and spiritual awakening. Founded in 1985 and located in Boulder, Colorado, we work with many of the leading spiritual teachers, thinkers, healers, and visionary artists of our time. We strive with every title to preserve the essential "living wisdom" of the author or artist. It is our goal to create products that not only provide information to a reader or listener, but that also embody the quality of a wisdom transmission.

For those seeking genuine transformation, Sounds True is your trusted partner. At SoundsTrue.com you will find a wealth of free resources to support your journey, including exclusive weekly audio interviews, free downloads, interactive learning tools, and other special savings on all our titles.

To learn more, please visit SoundsTrue.com/freegifts or call us toll-free at 800.333.9185.

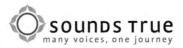